CUTTING LOOSE

A Biblical Approach to Health and Fitness

GILLIAN TAYLOR

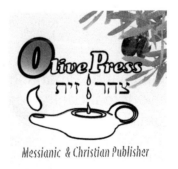

Messianic & Christian Publisher

CUTTING LOOSE *A Biblical Approach to Health and Fitness*

ISBN: 978-1-941173-20-6

Published by
Olive Press Messianic and Christian Publisher
olivepresspublisher.com
Printed in the USA

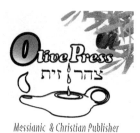

Messianic & Christian Publisher

Cover design by Karen Keene.

Interior design by the author and Olive Press.

Clipart images are copyright free from clipart.co.uk and bing.com/images.

Image on pg. 103 copyright © by Shutterstock.com. Used by permission.

Exercise photographs are the author's. All rights reserved.

NOTE: Having a British author and an American publisher, the choice was made to mainly use British grammar and spelling. For example: the British ending "-ise" vs American ending "-ize" and words like "whilst" vs "while," etc., were used to keep the author's British voice. American words are in parentheses when necessary for clarity. Some of the punctuation, however, is more American than British.

Author's website: www.christianhealthandfitnessfellowship.co.uk
Please get in touch with your feedback and questions:
CuttingLooseContact@gmail.com
The author is available for: Workshops, presentations, and talks.

Hear, Isra'el! ADONAI our God, ADONAI is one; 5 and you are to love ADONAI your God with all your heart, all your being and all your resources. 6 These words, which I am ordering you today, are to be on your heart; 7 and you are to teach them carefully to your children. You are to talk about them when you sit at home, when you are traveling on the road, when you lie down and when you get up. 8 Tie them on your hand as a sign, put them at the front of a headband around your forehead, 9 and write them on the door-frames of your house and on your gates.

Deuteronomy 6:4-9

Hebrew Names used in this book:

Hebrew	English
Yahweh	God
Adonai	Lord
Yeshua	Jesus
Mashiach (pronounced Ma-SHEE-akh)	Messiah
HaMashiach	the Messiah
Ruakh (also spelled Ruach) (ROO-akh	Spirit
Ruakh HaKodesh	the Holy Spirit
Tanakh (Ta-NAKH)	Old Testament

In this book, I will refer to Jesus as Yeshua because, quite simply, that is His original Name. I will be using Adonai for Lord and Ruakh HaKodesh for the Holy Spirit.

In the Hebrew language throughout the Scripture, God has many Names which describe His character and who He is. For the purposes of these studies, I will use Yahweh, the Name above all others.

CONTENTS

CONTENTS IN DETAIL

A Personal Message

Dear Friends in Yeshua HaMashiach (Jesus the Messiah),

You may wonder why I am opening this book about health and fitness with the passage from Deuteronomy. It is for me a plumb line and a constant reminder of the mighty and awesome God whom we serve. As we see the world turn its back on the One True God with mounting hatred, I believe that the time is short and that it is going to get increasingly harder to stand up for our faith.

We live in a world that is obsessed with the self, so if we too live this lifestyle, how can we have our eyes on our Creator God? How can we be living sacrifices? Where is our focus? If we are always tired, struggling to do our daily tasks, or if we dislike our bodies, how can we be living the life that we were created for? My prayer is that through these studies you will be able to see afresh and re-evaluate the uniqueness of His Creation in you and, by so doing, you can then begin to look at your own well-being from a new perspective.

This study book has been a long time coming, in fact, probably about seventeen years. Finally, it took a dear friend to tell me, in no uncertain terms, that if we have learned lessons along the way, then it is our responsibility to pass them on. Indeed, each one of you reading this will have gifts and knowledge that you need to pass on to others, in order to help them in their own spiritual walk.

There may also be those amongst you that do not have such a walk, that are perhaps confused or questioning the very existence of God, Yahweh. I am hoping that for you also, the following pages of study will help you towards finding the answers that you seek.

This manual is intended as a user-friendly study guide that will examine many health and well-being issues from a Biblical perspective. We rarely hear preaching aimed at our physical well-being. It might be argued that it is the spiritual that should have priority, and rightly so (1 Timothy 4:8). I am hoping, however, that through the following studies you will gain a better understanding of how inextricably linked the physical and spiritual are. I firmly believe that the time we have is getting shorter. The enemy is having a field day out there as he persuades us that we need to focus on self and that we are nothing unless we present with the perfect figure. Equally, we are living in a society that now accepts being unhealthily overweight and, conversely, underweight as the norm. Many of us are living a lifestyle that not only affects us physically in such areas as heart disease and high blood pressure, but that also influences our ways of thinking and how we perceive ourselves. Yahweh is deeply concerned with our wellbeing, spirit, soul, *and* body.

We will be looking in the first instance at some basic Biblical principles regarding health and well-being. It is the aim of these first studies to provide the reader with a sound Scriptural perspective from which to base the further studies. We will examine where we are, who we think we are, and where our focus should be. You need to take small steps, enjoy the studies, talk it out, walk it out, and enjoy fellowshipping together.

And most importantly…hold onto the truths that are in His Word.

My prayer for everyone is that we may be set apart, living apart, powerful, vital, allowing the Ruakh HaKodesh, the Holy Spirit, to govern our lives, to minister, to direct, and to guide. I pray that we can accept that we are wonderfully and awesomely made and that we can all be living our lives abundantly, just as our God, Yahweh, intended! (cf. Romans 12)

Yours in His infinite love,

Gill

Introduction

Welcome to *Cutting Loose*. This compilation of study material was never intended to be simply yet another diet and exercise book, but a study to offer a Hebraic Biblical perspective to health and well-being. I suggest that, unless we have a full understanding as to what is going on at a spiritual level, we will generally continue going around in circles.

We are awesomely made, unique, one of a kind, and made in His Image. We were created different sizes and shapes: some tall, some large, some small.

Questions:

- ❖ How should we view our physical wellbeing?

- ❖ Why do so many of us dislike ourselves?

- ❖ Does our physical wellbeing in any way affect our spiritual walk?

- ❖ Whose responsibility is it?

- ❖ Is it alright to resign ourselves to being overweight because "He made me this way"?

- ❖ If exercise "is not my thing" should I concern myself with it?

- ❖ Today we hear much about building self-esteem and confidence, but how do these fit with our spiritual walk?

I hope to respond, at least in part, to some of these issues. The studies will challenge and question what are often quite sensitive issues for many people. But most of all I pray they will inspire, encourage, and support you to make changes that will help you cut loose from the chains that can so easily bind us, so that you may live life to its fullest measure!

My intention is that the studies will help dispel many of the myths associated with health and fitness and identify some of the reasons we so often fail when we attempt to lose weight or improve our fitness. I also intend to give a new perspective to those of you who already enjoy keeping fit and healthy.

It is easy to get confused with the plethora of information on diet and exercise that is available. Without some basic knowledge, it is also easy to be conned into some rather extreme, frequently expensive, and often unhealthy practices that promise quick results. After the initial excitement of "this time it will work," motivation often wanes and many people fail to maintain what they had set out to achieve, which often results in a downward spiral of self loathing. These types of programmes are generally not focusing on changes to a healthy lifestyle, but rather on a feel good, quick fix.

What are the keys then to success and how do we stay motivated? How do we embrace a healthy lifestyle and how do we lose weight safely and effectively whilst walking strongly on our spiritual journey? We will be looking at all these practical aspects in Part Two. Of most importance is that we begin to understand the Biblical principles behind our approach to these issues and to establish the relationship with our spiritual walk.

I trust and pray that by bringing some of these matters to light, you will perhaps stand back from all you see and hear regarding all the pertinent issues, and reflect on the reality of what it is all about and how it affects you, the individual. It is about empowering you with the knowledge and expertise to enable you to make informed choices and changes and to build firm foundations on which you may stand.

Finally, let us look to Yahweh to instruct and teach. I am simply putting pen to paper and I ask that you test and approve everything that is written. There are no right or wrong answers to the questions I have asked, but I am hoping that the studies are sufficient to challenge and make you question and discuss the topics we will be looking at in a new and constructive way.

My people are destroyed for want of knowledge.
Hosea 4:6

But the Counselor, the Ruach HaKodesh, *whom the Father will send in my name, will teach you everything; that is, he will remind you of everything I have said to you.*
John 14:26

Preparations

PRAY!!

We will be looking at how to unravel the barriers that can so easily prevent you from living the life God intended, being free of the physical, mental, and practical things that may presently hold you captive. It is vital that we understand how our spiritual walk is connected with both our mental and physical well being, and it takes much effort and emotional strength to change behaviors of a lifetime. So please, it is vital that you spend time in individual prayer prior to starting these studies as well as before each meeting. Allow your Heavenly Father to prepare your heart and mind. Take hold in your heart that:

Therefore, there is no longer any condemnation awaiting those who are in union with the Messiah Yeshua. Why? Because the Torah *of the Spirit, which produces this life in union with Messiah Yeshua has set me free from the "torah" of sin and death*
Romans 8:1

The Studies

There are no hard and fast rules to the study elements, but the subject matter is designed to be read in sequence. It is, of course, entirely up to you, the reader, as to what you choose to follow. These studies are intended simply as a guide for an individual's journey in the company of friends. It is hoped that they will direct you, inform you, and help you to untangle some of the complex issues that we often experience regarding our health and well being, so that you may emerge stronger, wiser, and healthier.

There are numerous references given from Scripture. I have used the *Complete Jewish Bible* for no other reason than it is the one that I use most regularly. I have only identified the specific relevant verses within the studies, but I believe it is always a good idea to read the entire passage, if you have time, so that it is always in context. I do not think that it is particularly healthy, spiritually, if we simply pick out the verses that we like or think are appropriate. This is, however, my own personal opinion, so discuss this within your group and decide how you want to approach the readings and which version of the Bible you find most helpful.

It is also important to keep in mind that this book is compiled from my own experiences and studies on a spiritual, personal, and also professional level. They are not to be taken as the be all and end all, and you need to test and approve for yourself that which is written. Everyone reading this will have their own experiences and their own view on the Biblical interpretations. I believe that this is healthy and promotes a much deeper, 3D level of understanding. I cannot for one minute think that the disciples all sat around politely waiting to be invited to speak, not with their vibrant personalities and their passion. So, discuss these issues and bring your own ideas to the table. Be wise and use your discernment. Be involved, learn from each other, respect each others' views, and build on them, especially when you all disagree! This way, you end up with a wonderful, multifaceted diamond of knowledge instead of a flat piece of wood.

Study Groups

The following studies may well prove extremely challenging and will be dealing with subjects that, for many, are extremely sensitive. It is, therefore, important that you work through these pages with people whom you both trust and feel safe with. I would not advise large groups, maybe two to four, in order that you feel completely at ease at discussing some of the issues openly and honestly. Be involved, learn from each other, and respect each other's views.

It might be advantageous prior to starting, to decide who will lead each study. It could also be beneficial if this person reads through the next section to study in preparation. You may also like to consider discussing some guidelines, such as confidentiality. Sadly, in my own experience, with regard to what is often described by the term "sharing," things soon develop into something that is nothing short of gossip. So, please make sure that all of these issues are discussed openly and agreed upon. Keeping what is discussed between each other within the group environment will create greater trust and freedom. Please look out for each other and, if you feel it helpful, read through the following in preparation together:

- ❖ Support each other, the strong bearing the weak, **Romans 15:1-9.**
- ❖ Look out for each other, **1 Corinthians 10:24.**
- ❖ Uplift each other, **1 Corinthians 14:26.**
- ❖ Respect each other, **Romans 14:19-24.**
- ❖ We all have a part to play, **Ephesians 4: 11-23.**
- ❖ Love each other; respect each other, **Romans 12:10-21.**

    PLEASE BE SENSITIVE TO EACH OTHER'S NEEDS.

The Individual

For each and every one of you reading this, there is an amazing, unique life story. The *Cutting Loose* studies will mean different things to each individual. For some, it will simply be getting back into shape, easing back into an exercise regime, and getting back on track with a healthy lifestyle. For others, however, it may very well mean dealing with areas of your life that have held you captive for many years. I suggest at this stage that we need to be wise in these areas. In dealing with some of these issues, further professional help and expertise might be needed, such as a church counsellor or professionally qualified therapist. As an occupational therapist, I work within a team that may include: an acute clinical team, clinical trauma therapists, art therapists, mental health nurses, and specialist counsellors. There is absolutely no way I could, or indeed would, even consider being able to work independently. So, be wise, and, if appropriate, visit a suitably qualified individual or health professional.

If you entrust all you do to ADONAI, your plans will achieve success.
Proverbs 16:3

Summary

In summary, we shall be looking at:

Part One: Chasing Rainbows

Study 1 The Biblical Hebraic Perspective

This first study is to establish a clear understanding of the Biblical Hebraic perspective that underpins these studies. Not all who come across these studies will be living their lives from a Hebraic perspective and, for some of you, it may be the first time you have come across this point of view. So, this introductory chapter is by way of setting the foundations in place, to enable everyone to get the most out of the studies. We will be examining what is meant Hebraically by the physical body, the soul, and the spirit.

Study 2 Spirit, Soul, and Body

We will look deeper into what each of these entities are, how they relate, and how this impacts us. We may need to rethink our current understanding.

Study 3 Why Does Fitness Matter?

In this third study we will consider the balance between the physical and the spiritual and where our priorities should lie.

Study 4 What is Preventing Us From Living Our Spiritual Life to the Full?

We will focus on the issues that we are up against, not being fit. What are the areas that we have problems with?

Study 5 Where Do All These Issues Come From?

Where do we get these problems and barriers from? Is it simply the way we think? We will find out.

Study 6 How Do We Move Forward?

In the last study, we will consider how we are made in His image, fearfully and wonderfully, but also how easily this can be taken away from us, and how it can divert our focus away from Yeshua and our walk with Him.

Part Two: Firm Foundations

We will be applying the above knowledge to the practical hows and whys of a healthy lifestyle.

Lights
Knowledge through the Word

The studies will provide you with much information.

Write it down, talk it through, meditate on it, digest it.

Camera

Revelation, when He reveals understanding

Consider, meditate, dwell upon, pray about, and allow the Ruakh HaKodesh, the

Holy Spirit, to help you understand what He wants you to take on board.

Action

Our response

Part One

Chasing Rainbows

Study 1 The Biblical Hebraic Perspective

Introduction

You will need:

- o   Your Bible
- o   Notepad and pen

For some of you reading this, you may never have heard of a Hebraic perspective before, so let us very quickly summarize why we are using this as our foundation. I am no Biblical scholar nor an academic person, so the following explanation is quite simplistic.

Please read:

Genesis 12:1-2;   Exodus 6:6-8; 19:4-5

John 15:18-20; 17:15-16

Roman 12:1-2;   I Peter 2:4-5

Luke 2:22-24, 39, 41-42, 45-47; 4:16;

John 7:2, 10; Luke 14:12

Acts 3:1; 17:1-2

Acts 18:18; 21:23-24, 26; 24:14; 25:8; I Cor. 5:8

Consider this. Right from the beginning, we see that Yahweh (God) separated His people: Avram (Abraham), Noach (Noah), Yitz'chak (Isaac) and Ya'acov (Jacob). He separated Israel from the nations and brought them out of Egypt. Within the Brit Hadashah (New Testament), the term Gentile (which in those days would have been referring mostly to Romans and Greeks) is used to represent the world and its ways. We are not speaking in the sense of the country of Greece or city of Rome, but the way of thinking that the historical Greek and Roman cultures brought with them, as opposed to the Jewish way of thinking that Yeshua (Jesus) was born into. Yeshua asks us also to be separated, a people apart, to be in the world but not of it.

Yeshua was brought up in a Jewish household. We read that He attended Synagogue and listened to the Rabbis' teaching. He and His family celebrated the Feasts of Israel. The early church was predominately Jewish people who lived a Hebraic lifestyle, as we see in the verses given. You might say that Peter, after God showed him the sheet, stopped living Hebraicly. But the Biblical Hebraic Law never told the Jews not to go into Gentile homes. In fact, it says to love and be kind to the foreigner that lives among you (Deut. 10:19).

Why and how does this affect what we are studying now?

If we look at the history of the whole area around modern day Israel, the other Mediterranean countries, and beyond, we see that first the Greeks and then the Romans were in power over most of the region. Shaul (Paul) states that, within the Body of Believers there is no difference between Jew and Greek, but he also frequently had to teach how to overcome the differences that still existed in reality then and that still exist today.

The Greek, or Hellenistic, way of thinking effectively represents a Western mindset and, as such, most of us are influenced by it. Our whole way of thinking has been directed by Greek philosophers, such as Alexander the Great, Plato, Aristotle, and Socrates. It is these individuals who laid the foundations for our present day philosophy and psychology. Remember also that the Greeks, at the time, worshipped a plethora of gods (which the Romans also worshipped, but with different names), and Greek mythology is still studied in depth today. Consider how these many gods compare with the One true God: "*Hear, Israel! ADONAI our God, ADONAI is one*" (Deuteronomy 6:4 my paraphrase based on CJB), and we can already begin to see the differences emerging between Greek and Hebraic thinking. Sha'ul (Paul) frequently came across these differences way back then, and it remains the basis for our way of thinking in the West today.

Please read:

Act 17:29-31; 19:17-20

Phil. 3:19

I Cor. 2:4-5

Q. What conclusions can be drawn from the above passages?

Q. The Greeks worshipped the human body in the nude. God taught the Hebrews to never look on another's nakedness. How has this Greek thought affected our attitudes toward our bodies?

Q. The Greeks loved sports and competition, which was not part of the Hebrew culture at all. How does competitiveness maybe discourage your attitude toward getting healthy and fit?

We are about to look at the relationship between spirit, soul, and body, so we need to look first at each component and what Scripture tells us about it. We need to identify the differences between the Greek and Hebraic understanding of this subject and why it is so important that we approach this from a Biblical, Hebraic understanding.

In Greek thinking, the word for soul is transliterated as *psukh*, which is where we get our word psych from, as in the word "psychology." They considered man dualistic in nature, that is, there are just two elements that make up man. They believed that only the soul of man can be godly and that knowledge was key. The physical was considered as evil and, therefore, it was likely to do evil. The body was likely to do what came naturally to it, and, as only the soul would reap its after rewards, the body could do what it wanted to do. The soul was the most important part. If you now consider today's society, can you see how this way of thinking influences us?

Q. How have our society's Greek thinking sayings like "if it feels good, do it" or "how can it be wrong when it feels so right" affected your past behavior?

In contrast, the Hebrew understanding of the word soul, *nefesh*, embraces our whole being, not just our mind and emotions. It is the very gift of life, the breath and vibrancy of our body and our spiritual nature together as *one*—a *unit*—all embracing.

Yeshua identifies the greatest commandment for us:

You are to love ADONAI your God with all your heart with all your soul and with all your strength.
Mattityahu (Matthew) 22:37

And linked with this: You *are to love your neighbour as yourself.*
(verse 39)

If these are the cornerstones for our faith, and yet we cannot love ourselves nor grasp the fullness of who we are in Yeshua, our relationship with Yahweh will be limited, and it is doubtful that we could ever reach the fullness of life that He has created in us. If we remain influenced by this Western mindset, we are likely to struggle to come to terms with how our physical body can impact our spiritual walk. From a Hebraic perspective, it is imperative that we learn to consider our spirit, soul, and body as one entity, created as a whole in His likeness, that cannot be separated. What we do and think, how we speak and act, the decisions we make, the places we go, the lifestyle we choose are all intricately linked.

So, let us now move onto our first study and begin to apply this Hebraic perspective.

"The thief comes only in order to steal, kill and destroy;
I have come so that they may have life, life in its fullest measure."

John10:10

Study 2 Spirit, Soul, and Body

Introduction

You will need:

- o   Your Bible
- o   Notepad and pen
- o   Dictionary

In this second study, we are going to examine the relationship between spirit, soul, and body. Through understanding the complexity of this relationship from a Hebraic perspective, I hope that we may begin to see how our way of thinking and our physical wellbeing interact and how this influences our spiritual walk.

We need first to have a clearer picture of each of the parts that make up the whole.

Please read:

1 Timothy 4:8

1 Thessalonians 5:23

Hebrews 4:12

In the above passages, we see reference to three elements: spirit, soul, and body. The perfect balance to this is evident in our Lord Yeshua and in God the Father, God the Son, and the Ruakh HaKodesh. In the Tanakh, the Old Testament, we also see this reflected in the Tabernacle: the outer courts, the inner temple, and the Holy of Holies.

Discussion

You may wish to discuss this briefly and record pertinent points.

Let us now examine each of these a little closer.

The Body

In the above passage from Hebrews, we see reference to joints, marrow, and sinew—in other words, the physical body—but what else can we learn from Scripture?

Please read:

Genesis 2:7, 22

Genesis 3:19

1 Corinthians 3:16-17

Romans 6:12-13

2 Corinthians 4:7

Q. What conclusions can be drawn from the above passages?

Q. What functions does the physical body fulfill?

Q. How do the above passages describe the physical body?

Q. Can you accept that your physical body is God's temple and an instrument of righteousness?

Q. If you were in charge of the real Temple, how well would you look after it?
Would you maintain it, keep it clean, knock the cobwebs away, be protective over it, and consider it something special?

Discussion

We can see from the above passages that the body is made from dust and will return to dust, but what is its function?

We have, of course, all the intricate mechanisms that actually keep the physical body working. It keeps us in touch with the world around us, a world consciousness. We have our sense of touch, smell, taste, hearing, and sight. We can feel hot and cold. We hear the noise of a car approaching and the sound of birds. We see the flowers and trees, the garbage cans, and the graffiti. We taste bitter and sweet and can smell the freshly made bread. Our senses monitor everything around us, to keep us safe and to allow us to function physically. When someone loses any of their senses, they often find that other senses become heightened in order to compensate. Someone who is blind, for example, usually has very acute hearing and incredible touch sensation. Our physical bodies are amazingly intricate physiologically which we often take much for granted, usually until it goes wrong. The more I learn about the human body, the more overwhelmed I become by its awesome complexity. We are indeed created by a master craftsman!

Further to this, Scripture gives us a very clear picture of the physical body and its purpose. We see that we are dust and will return to dust: simple jars of clay, vessels, yet we were made in His image and are temples in which the Ruakh HaKodesh dwells. Here we are also warned about allowing sin to rule our mortal bodies.

Now if you re-read the passage from Romans 6:12-13

Q. Who is responsible for allowing sin to take hold?

Q. What happens if we allow this to happen?

IMPORTANT - Read: 1 Corinthians 6:19-20

KEY Q. What value does God put on you?

KEY Q. Does the way you think about your body agree with the value God has put on it?

   Q. Do you honour God with your body?

   Q. How well are you looking after your body?

The Soul

We have examined the difference between the Greek/Western thinking and the Hebraic understanding of soul. If you missed it, just quickly run through "Study 1 The Biblical Hebraic Perspective." We know that the Greek or Western understanding of soul, or psyche, is in reference to our minds, emotions, feelings, intellect, and our thought patterns. It is considered something that is separate from the physical. They equate the soul to our self will and our decision making process. The Hebraic understanding, meanwhile, encompasses all of this but also our whole being, the very essence of a person—the gift of life itself. This perspective draws the physical and spiritual together with the soul, the kind of closeness our Savior Yeshua, HaMashiach (the Messiah) has with the Father— they are one (John 10:30). We were, after all, created in His image.

Consider the following and look for the connections in the following passages:

KEY: If the will doesn't, the Spirit won't. We see this throughout Scripture.

Please read:

Luke 1:46-47

Psalm 34:1

Q. If then, the soul is responsible for decision making in the natural, how does it fit with our spiritual walk?

Discuss and reflect on how many times we are *asked* to invite Adonai in, to open our hearts. Knock and the door shall be opened unto you. Nothing happens without us making a decision about it.

Q. Is repentance an act of the will?

Q. Is forgiveness an act of the will?

Q. Where does self-dependence/independence fit in?

Q. Where does our choice/decision making, begin?

Read:

Matthew 22:37-40 (Cross reference to Deuteronomy 6:4)

Q. Are there any barriers you can think of that would prevent you from fulfilling these commandments?

Q. In summary, would you agree that the body fulfills the choice of the will?

Read:

Romans 8:5

Discussion

This intimate connection between our mind and body can be demonstrated in how we react when we are under what we perceive as a threat to our self. Think of an instance where you feel unsafe or threatened. Your body responds by going into what we call the fight or flight response. Your senses, sight or hearing, have seen or heard a threat. Your thought pattern perceives this, and a whole process of reactions are kick-started in nano seconds. Things begin happening beyond your control such as, your heart beat increases, you start to sweat, adrenalin is released, and your vision alters, to name but a few changes. All of this is for your survival so that you then have the ability to either stand and fight or run, but it wouldn't happen if there were no connection between the way you think—your mind—and your physical being.

The Spirit

If we consider the body as our world consciousness and the soul as our self-consciousness, then how can we describe the Spirit?

I think of it as our communion with Adonai, our God consciousness, our insight and discernment. We have already established that we are the temple of the Ruakh HaKodesh, the place of communion with God.

Please read:

Galatians 5:13; 16-26

Proverbs 20:27

Q. If the body fulfills the choice of the will, where does the spirit man fit in?

Please read:

1 Corinthians 2: 9-14

Romans 12:1-2

Q. When we consider now our physical and mental wellbeing, how should knowing the above influence our thinking?

Q. From where should we get our direction, influence, and strength?

Q. In the passage from Romans, how does it suggest we become transformed?

Discussion

If we are in any way cut off from this communion with the Ruakh HaKodesh by our own choice or by things that get in the way, are we simply operating from the soul? We can receive knowledge, but without the help of the Ruakh HaKodesh we cannot spiritually discern or understand, just like the seed that fell into shallow ground. Neither are we likely to make the right decisions, just like the seed that fell among thorns, and we will be open to anything the world teaches us.

How often do we see advertisements for mind and body days, or an evening with a psychic? These are clear examples of operating without Yahweh. Every person is made in His image, but if our spirit is dead to God, then it is liaising with a spirit world not of Yahweh's making, but through the soul, and we end up doing everything in our own strength, or soulishly.

Please read:

John 6:63

John 14:16

Galatians 5:24

And re-read John 10:10

❖ We have examined the wonders of His creation of us in His image.

❖ We have established that we are the Temple of the Holy Spirit and that He lives in us.

❖ We have also just established how intricately connected the spirit, soul, and body are.

Q. If our physical being fulfills the will and we have free will to make our own decisions, what influence should the spirit have?

Q. Could our physical wellbeing impact our spiritual walk?

Q. Should we care about our physical wellbeing?

Q. If so, how?

Q. Are there any areas that you can now identify physically where you might be being held back spiritually?

Q. With regard to your physical self, your perception of who you are, what you look like, and your health, from where should you seek direction?

Q. Are you doing all you can to maintain the health and well-being of the Temple?

KEY Q: From where do you seek direction?

KEY Q: Who/what influences you the most?

KEY Q: Are you Diagram A or B?

DIAGRAM A: In your own strength, from the soul.

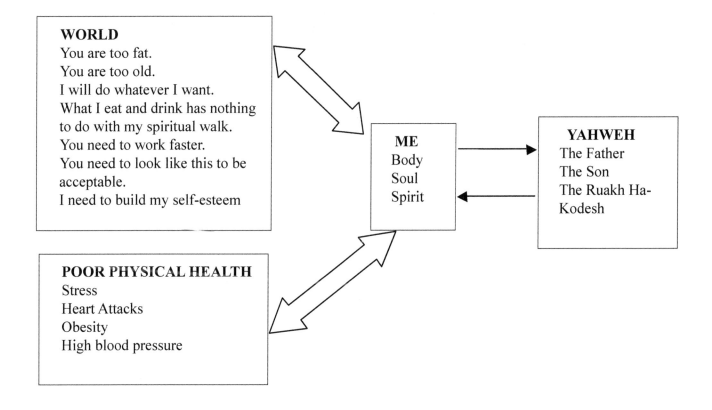

WORLD
You are too fat.
You are too old.
I will do whatever I want.
What I eat and drink has nothing to do with my spiritual walk.
You need to work faster.
You need to look like this to be acceptable.
I need to build my self-esteem

ME
Body
Soul
Spirit

YAHWEH
The Father
The Son
The Ruakh Ha-Kodesh

POOR PHYSICAL HEALTH
Stress
Heart Attacks
Obesity
High blood pressure

DIAGRAM B:

In His strength

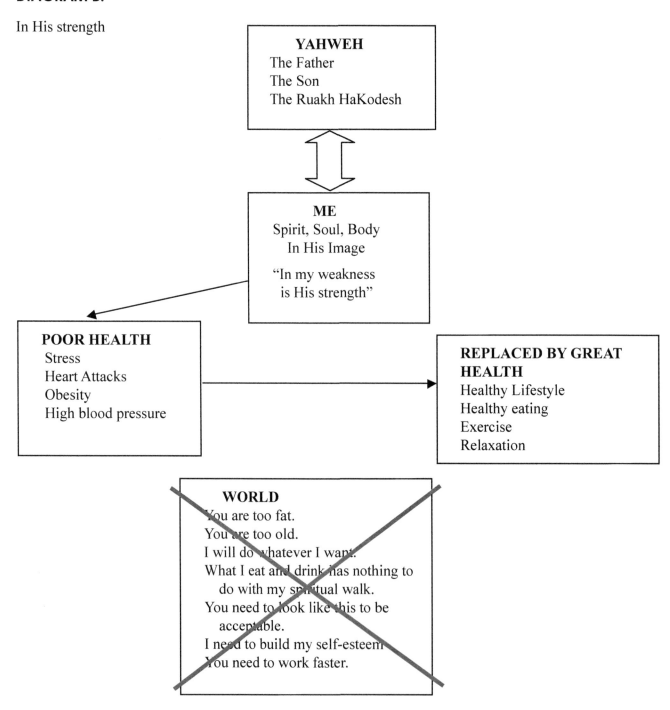

I am hoping that through these early studies you can begin to see how easily we can become distracted and frequently ignore our physical and mental wellbeing as something separated from our spiritual self. Let us now move on to think about why we need to consider possibly making some changes.

Pray for each other, that you may experience His Shalom as you move forward.

Study 3 Why Does Fitness Matter?

Does fitness *really* matter? Let us now look at why we should even be considering our health and fitness and hopefully answer a few fundamental questions.

Before we start this study, it might be helpful to discuss why you are actually thinking about taking this particular journey. You need to have it clear in your own mind why you feel you need to know more. It may be that after considering the following questions further, you choose not to continue, which is just fine, too.

I am presuming, however, that as you have chosen to look at the *Cutting Loose* course, there are issues that either interest you or cause you concern regarding your wellbeing.

Q. What is health / wellbeing? Establish what your group considers this to be.

Q. Using the knowledge from the previous studies, what attention should we be giving our physical and mental wellbeing, and how will this impact our spiritual health?

The secular view from the World Health Organization (WHO) says, *"Health is a state of complete physical, mental and social well-being and not merely the absence of disease or infirmity"*

(www.who.int/mediacentre/factsheets/fs220/en/).

There are endless consequences of neglecting our physical and mental health. We are continuously bombarded with health promotion: stop smoking, eat lean meat, eat more fibre, exercise more; so much so that I think we all perhaps become a little numb to it. Needless to say, unhealthy lifestyles with energy dense but nutrient low diets, smoking, lack of physical activity, and the stresses and strains of work or unemployment, together create a fairly toxic environment in which to exist. Added to this, to live as a Believer in Yeshua, to be in the world but not of it, and to uphold all the tenets of your faith is becoming ever more difficult in a world that is increasingly choosing to reject Yahweh.

Let's look at an example:

For an individual who is overweight and who smokes, the risk for associated illness increases dramatically:

- High blood pressure (Hypertension)

- Diabetes II

- Cardiovascular disease, such as blocked arteries and stroke

- Lung disease, such as Chronic Obstructive Pulmonary Disease and Asthma

- Joint disorders, such as lower back and knee pain and Osteoporosis

If we then also add into the mix how someone in this position may view and value themselves, we can quickly see how we can be robbed of so much physically, mentally, and more importantly, spiritually.

Please read and consider:

1 Timothy 4:7-10

1 Thessalonians 5:23

Romans 12:1-2

Consider:

Q. Where should our focus be?

Q. Where should our priorities lie?

Q. Should we completely ignore the physical?

Q. Who do you consider is responsible for your physical and mental health and well-being?

Q. What two things are we being urged to do in the passage from Romans?

Q. Do you consider your body as holy and pleasing to God?

Q. What issues for you, as an individual, prevent you from being able to accept this as true? (Maybe write them down.)

Q. Are we in any way conforming to the world? What does this mean?

Q. Should we be an example of living with self-control and discipline? Ouch!!!

Please read:

1 Chronicles 12:8

John 10:10

Q. When you look around your churches and fellowships, do you see a mighty army, fit for purpose and ready for battle, physically, spiritually, and emotionally?

Q. Are you living your life to its fullest measure in serving Yahweh?

Q. Can you accept that you are a beautiful, unique, one-of-a-kind creation, men and ladies?

Q. Are there any issues that are holding you back from experiencing all that Adonai has for you?

Q. Is your old self dead? Are you indeed a living sacrifice, poured out for Him?

I am hoping this study may have sparked some thoughts in your own mind as to where you personally stand, both on a practical secular level and also a spiritual one. It doesn't matter if you just have a few muddled thoughts at the moment. It may help to write it all down. It might be that you already have clarity on what concerns you about your physical self, so keep focused on these as we move on and try to apply the studies to your own situation.

May He bless you richly… … …

Study 4 What is Preventing Us from Living Our Spiritual Life to the Full?

It might be helpful if you just spend a few minutes reflecting and recapping on the first studies.

- What have you established so far through the studies?

- Are there any areas you need to look at more closely with the group?

- What balance should there be between your focus on your spiritual walk and that which you give to your physical and mental health?

- Do you think you personally have this balance correct?

We shall now explore this further with the aim of giving direction and focus.

You will need:

- Your Bible
- Large piece of paper
- Felt tip pens or similar
- Your own notebook and pen

Quick Quiz

Just to get you started, you may like to have a go at the following quiz. It is not necessary to discuss this with your group, but it may help get you focused. It is important that the issues you are up against are identified at the outset. Please be honest with yourself!!

1. In a few words try and describe yourself:

   How do you think others see you?

   How would you describe your personality?

   Identify what roles you have: mother, father, sister, uncle, welder, nurse, friend?

Who are you really?

2. How happy are you with your body? (Please check which apply.)

    o   I'm very happy with my body.

    o   I identify that He died for me and I am created in His image.

    o   I could do better, but I accept my body as it is.

    o   I dislike my physical body, but there is nothing I can do about it.

    o   I dislike my body and would do anything to change it.

3. Regarding the media, such as magazines and television programmes, how do you feel about
    the physical images that are portrayed, male and female?   (Please check.)

    o   I am comfortable with them and don't take them seriously.

    o   I never bother to look at them.

    o   I feel uncomfortable with them and avoid them if I can.

    o   I am concerned about the message they give out especially to youngsters.

    o   I think they set standards to aspire to.

    o   They make me feel unacceptable.

    o   They make me envious of others' lifestyles.

4. When I am over-stressed, I usually: (Please check all those that apply.)

- o   Comfort eat
- o   Treat myself and relax
- o   Pray about it
- o   Do some exercise
- o   Worry and feel ill
- o   Feel out of control
- o   Experience a low mood
- o   Go to bed
- o   Other

5. How do you feel when you are with your friends at a social event?

- o   I rarely go out.
- o   I always feel out of place and that everyone looks better than I do.
- o   I am comfortable with myself as long as I am with friends.
- o   I am really confident in who I am in Yeshua.
- o   I am usually the centre of attention.

6. How do you feel at church / fellowship?

- o   I always sit at the back. I have no skills that they could use.
- o   I offer to help if the opportunity arises.
- o   I would love to help and get more involved, but I don't feel qualified.
- o   I am always involved in something.
- o   I lead every group I can.
- o   I don't become involved due to restrictions from my medical condition.

7. Do you recognise areas that you would really like to change, or maybe ones that you have already tried to change? (Please check.) Please add your own as individuals or as a group. These are just examples.

- o   My weight is an issue for me.
- o   I would like to be more fit.

- I would like to improve on looking after mine and my family's health.

- I would like to complete everyday tasks more easily.

- I would like to be able to accept myself from a Biblical perspective.

- I would like to stop taking on the pressures that the world puts on me regarding my physical self.

Group Exercise

Using your large pieces of paper, spend a few minutes jotting down words and phrases describing all the issues that concern you. There are no right or wrong answers. Think of all the pressures that you feel you are under regarding your physical and mental well-being and how you feel and think about them. Try and include both individual and group experiences. If you have completed the quiz, perhaps use some of your answers to start the ideas flowing.

Q. What pressures have been identified?

Q. Are there common issues?

Q. What are we up against?

Q. Can you identify what might influence our way of thinking?

Q. Do your own feelings about yourself influence your behavior?

Q Does your weight and fitness level affect the way you perceive yourself in any way?

Q. Do you worry about your health?

Discussion

You may well be reading this and thinking, well actually, I am ok, and I really don't take on any of these issues. That is great to hear, but we should still be aware of how subtle the enemy is and also how our own thoughts can influence our behaviors. We can easily become entrenched in "acceptable" habits and behavior that become so familiar that we fail to scrutinize what we are doing. By way of example, an important issue that I have come across more frequently over the past few years is that of being **under** weight. This appears to be particularly evident in women and often with those who appear on the surface to have everything "under control." Frequently, this is accompanied with a recognizable unhealthy attitude towards exercise, which may be quite obsessive. This is influenced greatly by the celebrity lifestyle and has become increasingly acceptable.

While this appears to be more evident in females, one very important factor that tends to influence men to a greater extent is one of ambivalence, and especially to their health and weight. While these are just two very simple examples, I hope that it illustrates how easily we can be influenced without acknowledging unhealthy habits and lifestyles.

Constantly comparing ourselves with what the world decides is desirable will inevitably lead to such things as criticism and/or covetousness and frequently to self-condemnation.

Q. Are we communicating with a diminished sense of worth?

Q. Do we need to consider further our health and well-being?

Please read:

2 Peter 2:19

If you think it might be helpful, spend a few minutes just sharing with each other what you have learned as individuals so far. I am hoping that you have begun to have a clearer picture of where you find yourself and the issues that concern you, both as individuals and as a group. Remember, do not allow the things that might have come to light to condemn you in any way. We are to be in the world and not of it. I always think of the world as the farmyard. Even if you take extreme care walking through a farmyard, you will, inevitably, end up with a bit of mud on your boots. We just need to get the hosepipe out!

Before you close this session, read: **Romans 8**

Psalm 103

Home Study:

You might find it helpful at this stage to make a few of your own notes. Spend time privately with your Heavenly Father and allow the Ruakh to clarify things for you.

- o Try and identify what your own issues are.

- o Try and get a little closer to the cause. For example, comfort eating is not a problem, it is why you comfort eat that is the real issue.

- o Do you need to take your health and well-being more seriously? Do you need a health check? How is your blood pressure? What is your cholesterol level?

Once you have worked through these, spend time in prayer and allow the Ruakh HaKodesh to minister to you gently. Allow Him to reveal what you need to know and to help to identify some key issues that can be your focus for the following studies.

May He Bless you and keep you….

Study 5 Where Do All These Issues Come From?

Perhaps while the group arrives and you have your cups of tea and coffee, have a chat about what, if anything, you have considered this week in the light of the last study.

During your time of prayer, encourage each other, strengthen each other, and ask to come under His protection as you learn more. Guard your hearts and minds.

Please note: This is a lengthy study. If your time is limited, you may choose to split the study into more than one.

You will need:
- o   Your Bible
- o   Your own notepads and pens
- o   It will also be helpful to have a copy of a Dictionary.

In the last study we looked at some of the issues that might prevent us from living our lives to the full and in particular those that concern our health and well-being. In order to tackle these, we need to take on board our earlier learning: know where our focus is and from where we are seeking guidance. We need to try to place our health and well-being issues alongside our spiritual walk—in other words, keep a Biblical perspective. It might also be helpful to wise up to the bigger picture and acknowledge how the ways of the world can have an enormous impact on us as believers, if we allow it.

Please remember that as we explore these matters further, a number of you may well have been affected by really difficult issues. It is important that you allow your Heavenly Father to deal with these areas in your life in His way, in His timing, and when you yourself are ready, privately, gently and quietly. Please pray for wisdom in these matters.

Please read:

Ephesians 5:8-17

Ephesians 6:10-18

As you work through this study, try and bear in mind what these passages are suggesting we do. Keep it handy and re-read it, if necessary, along the way.

Q. What are these passages advising us to do?

Q. Why?

If we study the Tanakh/Old Testament we read repeatedly how the people of the time frequently turned their backs on God and were influenced by the society that they lived in. I wonder if this was always as clear-cut as we imagine. I contemplate as to whether this turning away was necessarily done intentionally, for want of a better word. I can just imagine how easy it would have been to have allowed the ways, beliefs, and customs of the peoples you were surrounded by to creep into your way of life.

Q. Do you think we live in such times now?

Q. What issues concern you as a believer about the society that we live in?

Q. Could the topics you considered in the last study be included in this?

Q. If not, where do you think they belong?

Q. Do we judge each other by the world's standards?

Q. Are we supposed to focus on self?

Discussion

Unfortunately, deception doesn't come with trumpet fanfares and all guns blazing. Rather, it is subtle, disingenuous, devious, and sly. Consider for a minute, expanding on all you discussed last week. If you have them on hand, use the answers from the quiz that you did in the last study and your collected ideas to stimulate discussion.

Perhaps you may like to discuss some of the following:

1. **Obesity rapidly increasing**   Around 1 in 4 people are now obese—leading to problems, such as heart disease, diabetes, and hypertension. Why?

2. **Eating disorders among the young**   Anorexia, Bulimia Nervosa, and Binge Eating Disorder are now evident amongst primary school children and rife amongst teenagers. Why?

3. **Personal disordered eating**   You are constantly thinking about what you can and cannot have to eat and are frequently dieting or bingeing. Why?

4. Poor body image common Out of all the clients I see, male and female, both as a health professional and a personal trainer, the majority dislike their bodies. This includes many wonderful Believers. Why?

5. Always considering *self*-esteem and *self*-confidence issues Why?

6. Plastic surgery common Why? (I refer to cosmetic surgery here, such as nose re-shaping, liposuction, or botox, not to plastic surgery necessary for medical reasons)

Q. Are these issues evident in your Church and Fellowship?

Q. Do you fall under any of the above headings?

Q. Do you consider yourself as unique in any way?

Q. Do you have a positive self-image of who you are in Yeshua?

Q. Is who you are in Adonai important, or is it more important as to how others see you?

Discussion

It is essential to acknowledge and to recognize where we personally stand. We need to know ourselves. Our thoughts generally determine our behavior and so without knowing the roots to our thoughts, behaviour, and understanding, it is difficult to tackle the issues that are keeping us captive. (See 2 Corinthians 10:5.)

In order to widen the picture even further, it might be helpful to consider the following subject areas and verses:

1. Materialism:

Mark 4:1-20 In the parable of the sower, many hear the message, but the worries of the world, the deceitful glamour of wealth, and all other kinds of desires push in and choke the message. So it produces nothing.

Matthew 6:24

Q. Do we actually have to have money to worship it? Why do we need a new car, a new mobile phone, and new kitchens? Do such items give us status and an identity? Do they help us to feel as if we belong?

Proverbs 21:17

Q. What do you think is meant by rich in this verse?

Ecclesiastes 5:9-11

Q. Does this apply to today's society?

2. Temptations:

The cultural temptations of the day influence us all.

> **Proverbs 23:19-21**
>
> **Proverbs 25:28**
>
> **Q.** Do we see and hear of these problems today?
>
> **Q.** Do we go for the "Meal deal" with extra fries or finish the packet of cookies because they are open?

3. Pride:

> **Ephesians 4:2**
>
> **Philippians 2:3-4**
>
> **Romans 12:16**
>
> **1 Corinthians 1:31**
>
> **Q.** Does today's focus on self contradict these verses?

Discussion

Does this mean we should all walk around in sackcloth and ashes and never have a treat or two? I don't think it does, but we do need to be on our guard and live, eat, and sleep in our spiritual armour. Scripture encourages us to be self-disciplined in all areas of our lives. Consider the subtleness of deception, something that is easily mistaken for the truth.

Proverbs 23:2

Romans 13:13-14
        6:12-14

2 Timothy 3:2

> **Q.** Is this true today?

2 Corinthians 4:4

> **Q.** What is meant by the spirit (god) of this age

What is:

- o Hedonism?
- o Humanism?
- o Secularism?
- o Narcissism?

Please read:

Ephesians 4:22-24

James 4:4

Q. Are we seduced in any way by the spirit (god) of this age?

Q. How do we know when we are loving the world without realising it?

Q. How should we respond?

Q. How does it affect our approach to health and fitness issues? From where should we seek direction?

Q. What does the passage from Ephesians advise us to do?

Q. How does Ephesians describe our new self?

Having now looked at the wider picture:

Q. Where do you think the issues that were discussed in the previous studies fit in?

Q. Where do you think the pressures you experience to be physically "acceptable" come from?

Q. Where does the ambivalence to our own health and well-being come from?

Q. Do you read the latest magazine and feel unacceptable?

Discussion

When you stand alone, and with nothing, before your God, who are you? Is what you have—your possessions—who you are, or is who you are in Him sufficient?

By way of an example, just consider for a minute what we know as the "celebrity lifestyle" and answer the following questions. (This is by no means a criticism of these people, but it may help to illustrate how easily we become entrenched in a way of thinking that then dictates our thoughts and behaviour.)

Q. Does this lifestyle have any influence on our lives today? If not on you personally, how about your children?

Q. What is their life based on?

Q. Do you read about their lifestyle? If so, how does it affect the way you feel about yourself?

Q. Why do we follow these "ideals"?

Q. If all these issues we have discussed above do not affect you directly, do they touch the lives of those around you?

Again, it might be helpful before you close to discuss what each of you has learned from this study.

Read together:

Psalm 4

Home Study:

It might be helpful to reflect on the above and in your own time consider:

- o   Where do you see yourself? Do you take what the world has to say on board?

- o   What influences your thinking?

- o   Do we take literally the instructions in all the Ephesians passages we've been studying?

Again, bring your concerns before your Heavenly Father. Ask Him to expand your understanding and to be able to see clearly what He would have you to know.

Read:

Numbers 6:24-26

Remember the value that God puts on you—He gave His Son!!!

Study 6 How Do We Move Forward?

In this study, we will consider how to apply what we have already learned. We will look more closely at how the body, soul, and spirit are connected and how this may directly affect our own perspectives. The aim will be to start re-evaluating our own outlook on how we both think and approach our physical and mental well-being and to study what the Scriptures have to say. It is intended that we will then be able to take this forward to the practicalities of our health and fitness program. This study is about drawing together all we have learned so far.

You will need:
- o   Your Bible
- o   Notepad and pen
- o   Sheet of paper from Exercise 1
- o   Large piece of paper and pen
- o   Dictionary

We have now established the difficult issues we may have regarding our physical self, how this affects the way we think about ourselves, and how it can impact our spiritual walk. We have also looked at the wider picture. It might be helpful to quickly reflect on what you have learned so far. Briefly jot down on your large piece of paper a few words that summarize the points we have looked at.

Here are a few questions to help you remember:

Q. What are the main issues that concern us about weight and self-esteem?

Q. Where should our focus be?

Q. On what do we base our ideas?

Q. Where do these come from?

Q. What is the spirit of this age?

Please read:

Genesis 1:21-31

Psalm 139:14

God made man in His image, and it was good. Furthermore, He had His hand on us before we were even thought of, each and every one of us.

It might be helpful at this stage to discuss these passages. Some people find it extremely difficult to accept these verses for themselves, that we are indeed "fearfully and wonderfully made." Somehow, we manage to dilute them to become more palatable, so read them again slowly and see what they say about you and I.

Our Greek society lacks the Hebrew culture of blessing our children. Therefore we may have genuine negative thoughts that can stem from childhood experiences, and these need to be handled with sensitivity. For example, if everything you have learned and experienced about yourself has been negative, then these will influence your core beliefs about yourself. We will be looking at this in more detail in Part Two, which I am hoping will complete the picture. In the meantime, it is important to support each other in prayer in these areas.

Please read:

Genesis 3:4-5

We need to consider here that the amazing truth was actually that we had already been created in His image and we are fearfully and wonderfully made.

Q. What does this verse indicate?

That the enemy is beginning his scheme to cause the Fall of man?

Q. Where is the enemy moving the focus to in this verse? God or self?

Please read:

1 John 3:8

Isaiah 45:22

Q. Does this reverse the Fall for those who are saved?

Q. Which way are you facing? Who or what are you looking to for direction?

Discussion

In light of the above about the creation of man, the enemy, and the Fall and together with all you have learned so far:

Q. What does "in His image" mean?

Q. Will the adversary be happy with this state of affairs?

Q. Will the adversary try everything in his power to destroy that image?

Q. Will he also try everything in his power to stop you living out God's purposes for your life?

Please read:

John 10:10

Q. How will the enemy do that? What will he use? Where will he find us most vulnerable?

Q. Does our own decision making process and free will also influence us, or create barriers to us moving on spiritually?

Q. Do you know what your purpose is for your life?

Q. Do you know what your identity is?

Q. Can you thank God for who you are, male or female, perfect in His sight?

Bear these points in mind as we move on. Try and apply them to yourself. I hope that you can begin to see that all we spoke about in the "Chasing Rainbows" studies can easily rob us of the promises that God has for us. You are awesomely and wonderfully made. You are precious in His sight. Your personality and everything about you is perfect for the life He has planned for you.

This study has been quite short, but I have left it so on purpose. I want you to really absorb what we have looked at here.

Finally, please read **Jeremiah 29:11-13** While in context this passage is speaking of Israel's exile, it contains some wonderful promises. We sometimes can also feel in exile, estranged, and an outsider.

Begin to hold onto some of these verses and memorise them.

Homework

In your quiet time, re-read the verses from this study, including and especially Jeremiah 29.

Praise the Lord that you are indeed fearfully and wonderfully made.

Read all of Psalm 139 and allow yourself to be immersed in His Word.

I am hoping that these few studies have helped to provide a clearer picture regarding the issues that you may be experiencing regarding your own health and well-being.

Keep a hold of everything you have learned so far as we now move on to look at how we can begin to embrace a healthier lifestyle. In Part Two, "Firm Foundations," we will look at just about everything you will need to achieve your health and fitness goals. Before taking the next step, perhaps you may like to spend time as a group praying for each other.

Please read:

2 Timothy 1:7

2 Corinthians 7:1

Part Two

Firm Foundations

Chapter One - Healthy Lifestyles - What are They and Why Do We Need One?

Consider Matthew 6:19-34

Spend time in prayer. Have a look around you at His amazing Creation, every tiny insect, every intricate flower, every bird in the sky, every majestic mountain and tree, the stars in the heavens and the waves that hit the shore…..you are a part of His Creation and you are so precious to Adonai, so precious that He gave His life for you. In our weakness is His strength, when we have nothing left, He can work in us. Focus your attention on pleasing Him and Him alone and be prepared to take a small step at a time. He *will* release you from the chains that bind….. He *will* cut you loose.

What is a Healthy Lifestyle?

For the purposes of this section, it is all about looking after yourself in the best way possible so that you can, in turn, honour Him. It is about looking after and feeding yourself correctly and about engaging in activities that you find **meaningful**, **purposeful,** and **enjoyable**. It is about reconsidering your body image and building your confidence in who you are as an individual, as you stand before your Master, Yeshua HaMashiach, perfectly created in Him. Keep hold of what we worked through in part one and focus on what you personally would like to work on.

Why is a Healthy Lifestyle Important?

In part one, we looked at whether or not we should be concerned about our physical well-being. Hopefully, you now have a clearer picture as to the "why" behind a healthier lifestyle, for all purposes, spiritual, physical, and mental. The flow chart on the next page illustrates it.

Unhealthy lifestyle / poor diet / little physical activity

Reduced motivation / poor self image

Reduced activities / increasing weight / health issues

Lack of confidence in who we are in Him/reduced motivation/no sense of competence/tiredness

Poorer physical health/hopelessness / lack of energy and vitality / self-loathing

We know that good physical fitness and a healthy diet reduces the risks of numerous diseases, including heart and lung disease, diabetes, obesity, some cancers, high blood pressure, to name but a few. Increasing amounts of evidence also suggest that the positive effects of good physical health is improved mental health. The UK government guidelines now recommend physical activity programs for most mental illnesses, including depression, anxiety, and stress related conditions. Improving both fitness levels and weight management strategies have also been found to have a huge impact on issues such as confidence, self-esteem, and self-efficacy as the world sees it, so it is also safe to say that this is also true as we build our confidence in who we are in Yeshua.

We have already established how intricately tied spirit, soul, and body are. So a healthy lifestyle, therefore, can go a long way to improving your mental and physical health, which in turn has a positive effect on the spiritual. The flow chart on the next page illustrates this.

Increased activity / improved nutrition

Improved mood / structure to the day / improved health

Improved sense of worthiness in Him
(He paid the ultimate price for us. That is the value He put on us.)

Learning new skills/new challenges/sense of achievement

Overall improvement in physical and mental health

Freedom from an unhealthy lifestyle and social ideals
Acceptance and confidence of who you are in Yeshua HaMashiach

Towards a Healthier Lifestyle

What do you need to change?

I have often been asked at what point should someone seek to make changes? If someone is quite happy as they are, then does that person need to think of making changes towards a healthier lifestyle? My answer is simply that when unhealthy behaviours impact your quality of life as a believer in Yeshua, then it is time to consider and pray about the need to change. Ask yourself, are you honouring God with your body? As the caretaker of the Temple of the Ruakh HaKodesh, are you doing the best job?

Make a General List

Don't think too much, just jot down any ideas. Focus on the areas that keep coming back to you and that really affect the way you are physically and psychologically. Discuss this with your group as there will probably be changes that you all agree on and you can then work together on them.

For example:

- o   Lose weight?
- o   Get more fit?
- o   Take more time to relax?
- o   Have a better balance between work and leisure?
- o   Eat more fruits and vegetables?

Stay Focused

Please read:

Matthew 6:33   *Seek Ye First*

Ephesians 2:1-10   *We are His workmanship*

Phillippians 4:13 – AMEN!!

Chapter Two – How Do I Start Making Changes?

All About Change

There is much written in the Scriptures about being pro-active when it comes to our spiritual walk. We are encouraged to run the race, work out our salvation, put in the effort, be determined, and to persevere. We have already established that our spiritual walk should be our priority, but if we also make the right choices in all things, and look after our physical and mental well-being, then we are surely pressing on to the very goal that the author of Philippians is referring to. In order to do this, we need to make choices and decide to commit to change.

The following texts are only snippets and it might be helpful to visit the relevant Scripture and to read it in full in context, discuss them in your groups, and then consider how to apply them.

Please read:

Philippians 3:12-21

1 Corinthians 9:24-27

Galatians 5:1-13

2 Peter 1:5-11

Discussion

Here the author is encouraging us to add to our faith, and then goes on to list all the attributes we should look to attaining, including self-control and knowledge. As in the above passages, these verses speak of adding these things through our own efforts.

How Do We Change Things?

It might be that you are quite happy and content with your physical and mental health as they are. If, however, you are not, and you feel ready to do something about it, then it is a good idea to actually establish why you are even thinking that you need to change, how ready you are to change, and what steps to take.

We must be careful not to be influenced by what the world considers behavioural theories, otherwise we are slipping back into psychology and a Greek mind set. There are, however, a number of practical observations that make perfect sense. So much so that there are a number of models that describe how we make changes. Have a look at the stages of change summarized here. See if you can identify where you are in the process.

Stage 1 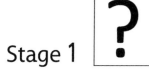 Contemplating

You are not ready yet to make any change. It might be that you are not yet absolutely convinced about the need for change. Your situation at present might prevent you getting to the starting blocks. You may have tried so hard in the past that you assume you will fail and the very thought of starting again makes you head for the biscuit tin, or is it the cookie jar….. Read on!

Stage 2 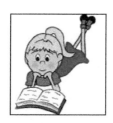 Incubating

You are thinking about doing something, but the next step seems too big or far away. You might not know where to start or how to take it forward.

Stage 3 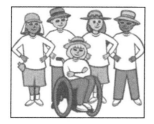 Preparing for action

Now you are beginning to focus on what you would like to do and how to go about it. Now is the time to plan and set goals.

Stage 4 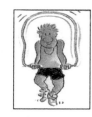 Taking Action

Your participation in making the changes has increased, for example, you are increasing your physical activity.

Stage 5 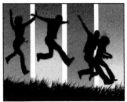 Maintaining

Now, looking after your physical and mental wellbeing is part of your lifestyle. It will require small changes to keep your interest and to keep you motivated.

Stage 6 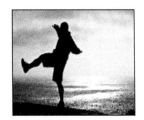 Oops, Things Not Going According to Plan?

This stage doesn't necessarily mean that you end up back at square one, or that you have to go through the entire process again. It might be, for example, that you are ill for a few weeks, the children are all on holiday, or that work is really hard going. When you can see the daylight again, you have already done the hard work, so you just have to decide how you are going to get back on track. Remember that you are aiming to change a lifestyle, thought patterns, and focus and all that will take time. You will have slack times and it is just as important that you learn how to flow with this. You need to learn how to rethink and make adjustments that will set you back in place. Even elite athletes have "off periods," and they certainly do not see it as failure, but rather as a time for rest and rebuilding. It is important to listen to your body. If you are ill, or busy, you may need a break…take one. Then, when you are feeling that you have the time and energy, you might need to revisit your original plan and re-set your goals. Remember that this is a change for life, not just a one hit wonder.

Once you have adopted positive healthy changes, keeping it up is much easier than you may think. If you take each step one at a time and gradually alter the things you do, the food you eat, the exercise you take, then slowly but surely you will notice the improvements for yourself.

The process of change tends to be cyclical in nature, which is great news, as it means if we go through a time where we are not really focusing, we can just get back on track when we are ready.

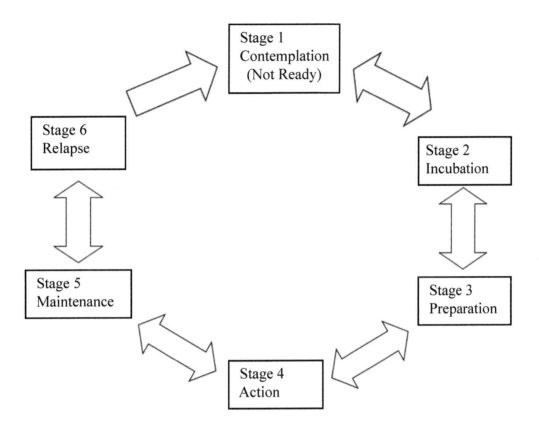

Have a look at the Decisional Balance Sheet on the next page, which you have probably seen many times before. If you think it is helpful, use the sheet and try and be as honest with yourself as possible. Using this will help you to identify where you are in the cycle of change. What are the pros and cons for you if you decide to change to a healthier lifestyle?

	Advantages for me	Disadvantages for me
Making Changes		
Not Making any Changes		

Putting It Into Practice

If you can understand how this process works, you will have a great tool when it comes to a healthier lifestyle. So, I really want you to come to grips with this and to understand exactly what happens when we undertake to change our behaviour. Remember that our thought processes influence our behaviour. The lifestyle behaviour we are presently leading is governed by what we choose, our decision making process, so remember what we discussed in part one about where our focus lies.

We will have learned certain behaviours from our parents and those around us. For example, if you were always fed fast food as a child, then the chances are you still eat them, or, if you were never encouraged to take physical activity as a child, then it is unlikely that you will participate now. Many unhealthy choices stem from both the way we were brought up and what is familiar to us. These choices easily become set in stone, and so often we never really give them a second thought. When we do try to change things, such as losing weight, we frequently take what is on offer, such as the latest diet, without really understanding why, what, or how this may or may not work.

Promises of losing several stone or kilos or pounds in a few weeks lures us to embrace the latest dieting trends. One guarantee is that you will lose weight if you stop eating! We cannot maintain this though, and so we then crave food, eat anything we can lay our hands on, and then assume we have failed. Making long term changes frequently requires changing behaviours that have become habits over many years and, therefore, you cannot expect it all to happen overnight. In setting a series of small goals and identifying less favourable habits, it is possible to really start to effect change for the long term.

The exercises on the following two pages may help you to focus on specific behaviours you might like to change.

Think of a behaviour or something that you would like to change. Try not to make it too drastic for now. Keep it fairly simple. It is amazing how small changes can make big differences. Changing behaviour is a skill, and as such requires practice, so start with manageable changes. For example:

- o Use less or no sugar in your tea or coffee.
- o Watch less TV and go out for a short walk.
- o Cook more meals from raw ingredients.
- o Start a new hobby.
- o Get to bed early.
- o   Pre-prepare a healthy lunch for work.

1. The behaviour I would like to change is:

2. Now try to think when the unhealthy behaviour started. Why are you not doing what you would like to?

3. Consider what is keeping you from doing this new behaviour and why you keep on doing the old one? What are the maintaining mechanisms?

4. Now complete the following table: the pros and cons to the current behaviour and any differences the change would make.

Current behaviour		If I change this behaviour	
Benefits	**Drawbacks**	**Benefits**	**Drawbacks**

5. On a scale of 1-10 how important is it that you make this change?

6. What might be the barriers to making this change?

7. What could you do to overcome these barriers?

8. Who will support you?

9. On a scale of 1-10, how confident are you that you can make this change?

10. On balance, do you think it is worth trying to make this change?

YES / NO

If the answer is no, move on!

If you answer no, then that is just fine…you are not ready to change this behaviour. Be happy with your current behaviour and move on. There will be something else to concentrate on that you will find easier to achieve. Don't waste time thinking about it any longer. Move away from the internal conflict. Focus on the positive changes that you have already made.

If the answer is yes, it is time to build your strategy.

You are now at a starting point and have achieved the first steps of your journey!!

You must now build your strategy for change. An action takes at least 15 repetitions before it becomes a habit. Studies suggest that 18 months is a good marker, after which a new behaviour will have become more or less established.

And Finally….

Take a **long term** view and remember that success is a journey, not a destination. Expect lapse, relapse, and even occasionally collapse to happen, and most importantly, accept that this is a normal part of the process of change. Don't just crumble into dust and grab the nearest muffin the first time something goes wrong. Have realistic sensible strategies for managing any lapses and getting back on track. Don't think that you have superhuman powers….no one else does!!

**IF YOU DO WHAT YOU'VE ALWAYS DONE,
YOU GET WHAT YOU'VE ALWAYS GOT!**
Henry Ford

Focus: Read Romans 8 and dwell on the richness of His promises to you. We are *more than* conquerors.

Chapter Three – Goal Setting

Remember Where Your Strength Comes From!

Read:

Proverbs 16:3

Changing behaviours and habits of a lifetime, especially when it is in relation to eating and activity, is difficult to implement and hard to maintain if you do not prepare and plan properly. Change may well upset the routine and sometimes it is easier to just live with what you know. The fear of failure often presents a huge barrier. One of the most valuable lessons an athlete will tell you, is how to learn from not achieving what you had planned—ordinary mortals would call it failure, whilst most athletes call these occasions building blocks. They will analyse them, reset goals, and set off again with a renewed vision. It is important, therefore, to set realistic, meaningful, and achievable goals as well as have contingency plans in place for when things don't go quite according to plan!

We need to narrow the viewpoint a little. It is too large a target and is open to failure if we simply state that we want to change to a healthier lifestyle. We also need to grade what we hope to achieve. When climbers attempt to reach the top of a high mountain, they do not just set out for a hike and expect to get to the summit in one go. The routes are planned in infinite detail and a series of camps set up to split the route into achievable sections. This does not diminish their achievements in any way. Indeed, good planning is part of that achievement.

So we need to:

- ✓ Identify the end goal.
- ✓ Split the route to that goal into achievable portions.
- ✓ Set mini goals along the way.
- ✓ Identify possible barriers.
- ✓ Have a strategy in place for when things go off track.
- ✓ Identify a trustworthy support network.

Before starting to plan your goals, it is helpful to identify what your priorities and values are and to get some ideas going. Your goals need to be meaningful to you as an individual. If they are not, and you are just doing it because you feel you need to, then you are unlikely to be successful.

    ✓ Consider carefully how and what you set as your goals…..be inspired and keep them exciting.

    ✓ Discuss all your goals within the group and bounce ideas off each other.

Here are five steps you might find helpful.

Identifying Goals….

Step 1

List as many things that you can think of that you value with regard to your health and fitness:

Step 2

Now list the 10 most important of these in order of priority:

1._____   6. _____

2._____   7. _____

3._____   8. _____

4._____   9. _____

5._____   10. _____

Step 3

Choose one to work with and to set goals from, BUT make sure it is a realistic one and not just wishful thinking.

Step 4

Jot down your likes and dislikes as regards areas that will influence your goal setting.

For example, its no good including swimming in your activity schedule if you hate the water! BUT, if you love walking then this may be the very key to increasing your levels of physical activity every day.

Likes: Dislikes:

_____   _____

_____   _____

_____   _____

_____   _____

_____   _____

Step 5 –A KEY to Success…. Charity Challenges

One way of choosing goals, for both increasing physical activity and healthy eating, and one that I have found unendingly successful, is to get my clients to think of a challenge that they have always wanted to do, but never dreamt possible, that is part of a charity event. If you find yourself a charity challenge, you will have a set date and a focus and a commitment to improve your fitness level, and it will be for a great cause that you feel strongly about. Again, be realistic, but also don't limit yourself. You could do a local sponsored walk, a marathon swim, walking up a mountain etc. If you are working this out on your own, it is a brilliant way of making new friends too. Lifelong friends are frequently forged amongst all the sweat and tears!

In England, we have an annual 5K run series for a women's cancer charity. This annual race has probably achieved more success in terms of getting ladies out training, than all the health clubs put together! It is fantastic fun with amazing camaraderie, and it raises millions in funds. You know when it is coming up because you see groups of ladies out jogging, power walking, and running *everywhere* and you have to wear pink! It is so good to see.

Doing a challenge for someone or something else takes the focus off you, and you will now be doing something really worthwhile, as well as changing unhealthy behaviours for yourself. Focusing on who you are doing it for makes the doing of it so much more meaningful and, of course, it is raising much needed funds for the charity. This, coupled with the sense of achievement that you experience at the end of these events, frequently changes the participant's perspectives for life. Training for a charity event and setting it as a goal also makes the times where it gets a bit tough going much easier. When you begin to feel sorry for yourself and the last thing you feel like is going out power walking in the rain, or getting your push bike out, then all you have to do is think of the people you are doing your challenge for, and the motivation will simply generate itself.

There are hundreds of fabulous events both in this country and internationally that are worth looking into. If you have access to the internet, have a search around your favourite charity site. If you don't, then approach the charity directly and ask them for the relevant information. I have had clients cycle across Cuba, climb Kilimanjaro, cross the Sahara, walk up Ben Nevis, do local sponsored cycle rides, and sponsored swims, in other words, all sorts. If you are less able, don't tell yourself you can't be involved, simply get your thinking cap on and choose something that you are capable of doing. I have a number of friends with Multiple Sclerosis, and together they did a sponsored swim, a relay event, with the more able bodied of us doing a few laps when they were feeling too fatigued. It was huge fun and raised a considerable amount for the local MS charity. We also had a very nice, well deserved meal out afterwards! I also now work with disabled Veterans….you *can not* tell them they can't do something….be inspired!! You need to find an event that will take you out of your comfort zone, that you can get excited about. Focus on it, get your friends involved, possibly do as a church/ fellowship together, commit to it, and, if you can't find one, organise one…..ENJOY!!!

Our charity challenge this year will be:

.

Now that you have a better idea of what goals you wish to set, you need to make these into what are called SMARTT goals.

Setting S.M.A.R.T. T. Goals

You may well be familiar with SMARTT goal setting. Setting SMARTT goals is key to the success of your programme. It is about planning and preparation and about providing a solid foundation from which to work. I usually add an extra "T" for Time Out.

SPECIFIC: Write down *exactly* what it is I want to achieve.

MEASURABLE: How will I know when I have achieved this goal?

ACHIEVABLE: How am I going to achieve my goal? Is it achievable?

REALISTIC: Is my goal realistic? Every goal we set, especially in health and fitness, needs to be realistic. It is quite feasible to set high, long term goals, but we need to break them down sufficiently into plenty of shorter term goals that provide a series of stepping stones to our final target.

TIMED: When do I plan to reach this goal? Having a timescale really helps to set strict guidelines.

TIME OUT: What happens if something prevents me from achieving this goal in the time I have set, or what happens if I have a few weeks of ill health? It is good to have contingency plans. No athlete trains consistently without set backs, and it is the same for everyone else. It might be that you just need to reset goals and readjust the timing. Remember that the *Cutting Loose* programme is all about **long term** changes and so you have to allow for times when things don't go according to plan. The *KEY* is allowing for these times and writing it into the whole programme. It is recognising that no one can train 24/7 successfully. It is learning to pick up where you left off *WITHOUT* thinking or imagining that you have failed in any way.

More About Setting S.M.A.R.T.T. Goals

They need to be broken down into:

1. Long Term Goals: I usually look at 6 months for my clients. Any longer than this and it is difficult to visualise, and any shorter is far too pressurised.

For example: To have lost 2 stone (28 pounds) in weight

2. Medium Term Goals: I usually split this at 4 months.

For example: To have lost 1 ½ stone (21 pounds)

3. Short Term Goals: Now here is where I continue to split the target goals down – in order to achieve my longer term goals.

Weeks	Target weight loss
1-2	1-2 lbs loss
4	4-5 lbs loss
6	6-7 lbs loss
12	8-10 lbs loss

Then, at 6 months, I would review the goals with the client and look to the next 6 months, so maybe another 28 pounds if there was that to lose. If I had suggested initially to lose 4 stone (56 pounds) in 12 months, it could have been too overwhelming when first starting out.

In this example of weight loss, I would be quite specific and state exactly what and how I hope to achieve my client's targets. All this goes into the goal-setting schedule as a daily diary for my client to follow. I will also document the physical activity programme and detail the healthy eating schedule.

We will be looking at physical activity and healthy eating programmes in more detail in later chapters, but remember the more you plan, the easier it will be simply to follow your own guidelines.

Set **Specific** goals	Rather than **Vague** goals
By April I will be walking to work three times a week. I am going to join the local sponsored walk for charity in six months time.	My goal is to get really fit.
I want to lose a stone (14 lbs.) by my birthday in six months time.	I want to lose weight.
I am going to swim every Monday starting this week.	I am going to start swimming.

Further Instructions for S.M.A.R.T.T. Planning

Example Goal: Learning to swim through swimming lessons

SPECIFIC: Write down *exactly* what it is you want to achieve. For example:

I want to learn to swim is alright BUT

What do you specifically want to do –

a. Swim in the Olympics

b. Swim across the local pool

c. Feel safer in the water

MEASURABLE: How will you know when you have achieved this? For example:

a. I have an Olympic medal.

b. I have reached the other side by swimming.

c. I feel confident now in the water.

ACHIEVABLE: How am I going to achieve my goal?

Break it down into smaller steps.

In this case, the swimming teacher will already know what stages to take you through, but it will help if you see those small steps yourself.

For example: My feet no longer touch the bottom when I swim.

REALISTIC: As we have already discussed, every goal we set, especially in health and fitness, needs to be realistic. It is quite feasible to set high long term goals, but we need to break them down sufficiently into plenty of shorter term goals. The above example is perfect. Learning to swim is a significant challenge but very achievable when broken into smaller steps.

TIMED: In this example it is a course over a series of weeks, so that is already decided.

TIME OUT: If I need to, I can take time out and then rejoin the next course.

And finally ……Tips to Manage Relapse

Think about likely causes that may steer you away from your plan. This is about looking at possible situations that will draw your focus away from your programme. If you are working through this with friends, or as a group, have a chat about what you think may get in the way of you progressing, and write them down. In the groups I have run, we have had all sorts of issues that can flash up as barriers, here are a few:

- I feel guilty when I take time for myself.
- I always have to eat everything on my plate.
- The packet of biscuits was open, so I had to finish them.
- My children always want fast food.
- I am too tired when I get home from work to do anything other than watch television. ·

If you were to now go through this list and mark those that you could actually change or control if you wanted to, it will give you a new perspective. So, be honest with yourself and don't make excuses!

It is about all the things that you can find solutions for if you put your mind to it. These can be incorporated into your SMARTT goals. The advantages of working this programme through in a group is that you can pick each other up when you are finding it difficult…….AND don't forget to pray about it!

On the next page are a few examples of addressing the potential pitfalls.

Common Situations	Practical Solutions
Family or Time pressures	✓ Get the support of a friend or family member to make sure you allow time for your programme. ✓ Prioritise all jobs and ensure that you create "guilt free" time for your programme. ✓ Remember that you are responsible for your children's health and well being and to give in to the pressures of them wanting unhealthy foods isn't necessarily the best route.
Less active	✓ Get out for a short walk. ✓ Walk or cycle to work. ✓ Plan your day to include physical activity. ✓ If you drive a lot, take fruit and low calorie snacks with you instead of fizzy drinks and sweets. ✓ Take the stairs instead of the escalator
Social pressures	✓ Enjoy high fat foods occasionally and then get straight back on track. ✓ Eating out: opt for lower fat dishes.
Living alone	✓ Check labels before buying ready meals. ✓ Don't buy all your comfort foods. ✓ Choose low fat options. ✓ Have a supply of baked beans, tuna, pasta, low fat sauces. ✓ Eat regularly. Try not to skip meals, especially breakfast. ✓ Cook proper meals for yourself. ✓ Try a new hobby. ✓ Join a local group. ✓ Get your friends to walk with you.

Have a look at the suggestion below. It is taken from a personal health plan diary. I always encourage my clients to write down as much as possible. So, if you think it might help, get yourselves a little diary and put all your ideas down. This way, you can keep referring back to it, and you can keep checking on how you are doing. In later chapters, I will mention both Truth diaries and Training diaries, which you may also find helpful. The majority of people forget where they started and how well they are doing, so it's good to record it on paper. Some people keep all the diaries as one. Either way, feedback from most people is that once they have learned to use them, they report that they become invaluable and help to keep them on track.

My Healthy Lifestyle Diary

My first S.M.A.R.T.T. goal is:

What am I going to do to help me achieve my goal?

Where?

When?

Who will support me?

How will I know how I am doing?

What will I record?

When will I record?

Barriers:
Places and things that make this programme
difficult:

People who make this programme difficult:

Thoughts and feelings that make this programme
difficult:

Practical Solutions:
Places and things that make me feel
comfortable:

People who will help me:

Thoughts and feelings that make it easier to do
this programme:

Consider what you have read and worked through in this chapter. Now pray it through and

give these ideas back to Adonai. May He richly bless you as you trust Him and step out in His strength.

Chapter Four – Take Time Out

You will hopefully now have set your goals and have a clearer picture of where you want to get to and how you are going to achieve it. It might be helpful to take some moments to read through and dwell on the verses below before moving on any further.

We all know how frantically busy we all are. Most of us are juggling raising a family with highly pressurised jobs and the demands of earning enough to make ends meet. Some of you reading this may be managing long term ill health or be unemployed which can, in themselves, create vast amounts of stress. When individuals commit to get fit and move towards a healthier lifestyle, they frequently put themselves under enormous amounts of pressure to achieve what are, quite often, unrealistic goals. The *Cutting Loose* programme is about adopting a healthy lifestyle for life. So you have, effectively, the rest of your life to work at it. This programme, therefore, is not about adding to the demands that are made on you already, but more about gaining strength for the task ahead. It is about renewal, especially of your mind, refreshment, restoration, and rebuilding. Reflect on what we looked at in Part One, **Romans: 12:1-2.**

So, when you now start your programme, remember to keep your eyes focused on Yeshua. It is no longer about you struggling to lose weight, or to eat properly, or to exercise more; it is more about refining your spiritual walk by improving both yours and your family's health and well-being at whatever level you can achieve, gradually and effectively.

The definition of "rest" is all about having time and space away from the normal hustle and bustle. We read often about "rest" in the Scriptures.

Please read:

Mark 6:30-31

Hebrews 4   (about the importance of taking a Sabbath, a day of rest)

Q. Does your Sabbath exist?

Do you ever have a time where you switch off the television, mobile phones, and the computers? Do you spend time with the family and resting in the shadow of His wings, or is your life an endless round of catch up, meeting deadlines for the boss, or keeping up with looking after a family. On your Sabbath day, do you frantically scramble around to get off to your fellowship meetings as if it were another school day? Do you strive to meet your own itinerary when it comes to your quiet time? Does your Bible study leave you exhausted? When do you have me and Yahweh time? When do you just stop and wander around the garden, or round the local park just taking in His creation, with no mobile on, no talking, no distractions? When was the last time you simply stopped and allowed your Heavenly Father to get a word in?

Have a look at the dictionary definitions for

Restore:

Renewal:

Please read:

Psalm 51:10-12 (Perhaps you could use this as a prayer.)

Isaiah 40: 25-31

Just dwell on these for a moment. If you are working through this with others, have a chat about their relevance.

Q. Do you think that these apply to what you are doing?

Q. When was the last time you looked at the clouds, or took time to look at the stars, walked through a garden and knelt to smell the roses, watched the trees toss in the breeze or the waves on the shore? Yahweh who created these, is this the same One that cares about you and what you do?

Beware, however, the current upsurge of "meditation" and contemplative prayer where one is encouraged to empty the mind. We are instructed to wear the full armour of God and to meditate on His Word, not to replicate New Age practices by striving for altered states of consciousness. In the UK these practices are becoming common place in our churches and we need to wise up to deceptive practices.

To check this out, read:

Joshua 1:8

Psalm 1:2

Philippians 4:8

Consider **Isaiah 40:30-31**

Q. Are we expected to fall at some stage, get weary? What is the answer?

- o When the weight isn't coming off as you expected

- o When your boss is on your case wanting deadlines to be met and you know you are overeating

- o When you get so tied up with family commitments that you haven't had a minute to yourself

- o When you worry about your health

- o When you feel like giving up

What is the answer?

Q. Do you remember the hour you first believed?

Please read:

Psalm 51

Colossians 3:10

Titus 3:4-7

I am hoping that by studying these few Scriptures, you can approach your goals from a perspective of renewal. See it as rebuilding and restoration. We looked at the physical body in Part One where we saw it described as the Temple of the Holy Spirit. For further reading have a look at how many times the Temple was cleansed and restored in the Old Testament such as in **1 Kings 15:12; 2 Chron. 15:8; 29; 33:16; 34:8-14**. Then after the Temple was completely destroyed by Nebucadnezzar, read about the restoration of the walls of Jerusalem and the rebuilding of a new Temple that are so beautifully described in **Nehemiah** and **Ezra**. Whenever this happened it was done with dedication, loving care, obedience, planning, and in His strength….. Hallelujah!

Chapter Five – Healthy Eating

Introduction

Genesis 9:3

Genesis 3:19

So Keep It Simple and Eat What You Grow!?

The following chapters are meant as something of an introduction to healthy eating and weight loss. For each person reading this, your knowledge about the subject will vary greatly. I am not a specialist, dietician, nor a nutritionist, so the information provided is basic and user friendly. I have documented all the methods and knowledge I use as a health professional and personal trainer in both my weight management classes and when working with individuals. It is what I have found works over the years, that also embraces all the current guidelines from research and is that which constitutes a healthy eating plan.

It is easy to become overwhelmed and confused by the amount of information that is out there. Every week there seems to be some new piece of research that changes current thinking, so I will outline some very simple guidelines that I am hoping will make your healthy eating simplistic and easy to adhere to for both you and the people you care for. Long-term weight loss should be *achievable without heartache*, and I hope the following chapters provide a simplistic, flexible, and workable model from which to work.

Before you start the next few chapters, it would be helpful to complete the following worksheet. Keep this on hand so that you can refer to it as we move through the chapters.

Healthy Eating Checklist

This is just a very quick checklist. So don't spend hours on it. We will use it to see how much and what you need to change. Frequently, making a few small changes can make a very big difference.

What do I eat and drink at these meals? *Jot down the foods and drink that you consume regularly*				
Breakfast	*Lunch*	*Dinner/Tea/Snack*	*Supper*	*Snacks*

What meals do I eat each day?   **Please mark all that apply:**

☐ **Breakfast**

☐ **Lunch**

☐ **Dinner/Tea/Snack**

☐ **Supper**

☐ **Snacks sometimes**

☐ **Snacks instead of a proper meal**

☐ **Snacks all the time as well as meals**

☐ **Sugary drinks (including alcohol)**

What is Healthy Eating?

We hear the phrase bandied around all the time, but what does it actually mean on the plate? Here are some of the responses given in my local weight management classes:

o   Five a day (fruit and vegetables)

o   Lettuce leaves!

o   Watching what you eat

o   No chocolate

o   Rabbit food

o   Organic foods

o   Diets

It is interesting, though, that as soon as you mention healthy eating, most people associate it with words like "control" and "boring." Healthy eating is something everyone should consider and is about giving your physical body the correct nutrient rich foods that it needs to perform at its best. Healthy eating is not about control and neither does it need to be boring, rather it is about choosing healthy options. It may well involve changing from eating take outs to home cooked meals, but that lends itself to being creative and imaginative around your food. It is also about planning and taking care that you feed yourself correctly instead of running out of the office or stopping your car to grab the nearest pastry or burger.

Of most importance, healthy eating is also about feeling comfortable around food and allowing yourself the freedom to enjoy what Yahweh has provided.

Our physical bodies require certain amounts of specific foodstuffs in order to operate effectively. If we do not feed it the correct foodstuffs, or indeed overfeed it the wrong foodstuffs, there are consequences. It is as simple as putting diesel in a petrol (gasoline) car…it will break down.

Information can be extremely confusing. For example, most people had come to appreciate that overeating foods high in saturated fats, such as deep fried foods, fast foods, and pastries, etc., may clog up your blood vessels, which puts you at a much greater risk for problems like a heart attack or a stroke. Current findings, however, suggest that this may not necessarily be the case and that it is sugar that is the real bad boy.

You can get very tied up with all this. So, what I would suggest is that you use the following key points and find what works best for you and your family:

1. Eat in moderation

2. Cut portion size down

3. Eat plenty of fruit and vegetables

4. Limit products with both sugar and high amounts of fat

5. Up the physical activity

6. Drink plenty of water and cut the sodas.

7. Do you feel well and have enough energy? If not, try some changes to your diet. It might be that you have too few carbohydrates, not enough protein, or are eating foods that are unsuitable.

8. Don't be extreme, the dieting industry is based around you failing....it is worth billions!

Likewise, if we miss certain foodstuffs, then there are equally significant consequences. A current example is the prevalence of Osteoporosis, due in part to a lack of calcium in the diet. In Osteoporosis, your bones become extremely brittle and effectively your skeleton is no longer able to support you properly. It is generally characterised by frequent fractures of the skeletal bones. If you consider that an entire generation is growing up on a diet of products such as fizzy drinks rather than milk, then the picture is not very rosy for the future as this illness goes. Weight bearing exercise is also important to build strong bones, and the current lack of physical activity in people's lives exacerbates greatly the risks of developing this debilitating disease.

Quick check;

Q. Have a quick look at your checklist. Do you eat a lot of high fat/high sugar foods?

Q. How many fizzy/sugary drinks do you have in a day?

So What is a Nutrient?

A nutrient is what the body needs to work, such as: carbohydrates, proteins, fats, *yes fats*, vitamins, and minerals, as well as plenty of water.

How Do I Eat More Healthily?

Think for a minute of that which our Heavenly Father has provided for us: we have meat, fish, beans, nuts, and dairy for our protein requirements; all the grains for our principle carbohydrate and energy needs; oils and fats that are necessary for our bodies to function; and, finally, fruit and vegetables, nuts, beans, and seeds that both compliment the above and also complete our mineral and vitamin requirements. Take an orange for example: it comes in its own neat little packaging, bright and attractive. Most people know that oranges are a good source of Vitamin C. We need Vitamin C for maintenance of a number of our body's functions, including our bones, teeth and gums, blood vessels, and our immune system—to fight off infection. Oranges also contain the important Vitamins A, B1, B2, Niacin, Folate, B6, and Vitamin E, as well as many of the minerals that we need. In brief, what Creation provides is exactly what our physical bodies require to work properly, and it is to these that we should be looking for our nutrition.

Healthy Eating is Based On:

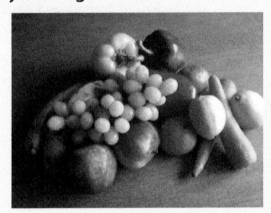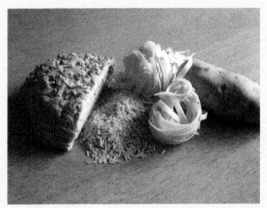

Abundant fresh fruit and vegetables …Good oils such as olive oil…… Nuts and seeds…...
Fish and lean meat…. Complex carbohydrates such as wholegrains……Moderation and portion control

Today, we are faced with vast amounts of processed foodstuffs that are frequently not only high in fat and sugar but also are of very little nutritive value, that is, they do not supply anything that the body really needs. High levels of both fat and sugar create enormous problems for our bodies and results in further issues like obesity and diabetes as well as those that have already been discussed. Unfortunately, we also enjoy these foods and easily become accustomed to the taste of high fat and high sugar content, for example, fat adds to the "mouthiness" (fullness) and flavour of food. But once you are aware of what nutritive value (or lack of value) foodstuffs have and exactly what we need to remain healthy, then you can make healthier selections.

Before going further, I would like to briefly consider a few comments that are frequently made when healthy eating is discussed, as they can often become barriers to making healthy changes.

o   It is expensive

o   My children won't eat it

With the advent of cheaper supermarkets (in the UK, especially), the foodstuffs we are talking about are now cheaper. Fruits and vegetables from these outlets are generally of a high quality as are the cheaper cuts of meat. These shops are now reasonably widespread. (We even have one in my little town in Yorkshire!) There are also local markets of home-grown produce that are now becoming more widely available, and you could also grow your own. In the cities, the ordinary supermarkets do now have what is usually a basic range of fruits and vegetables.

High fat/high sugar foodstuffs can be almost addictive as well as bad for our health, and it is important to consider what we are feeding our family. I do not have children, just buckets of nephews and nieces, so I am really in no position to comment, but when I talk with Mums and Dads, they do agree on the following. When it comes to the children, what they eat and how healthy they are is your responsibility, not theirs. Childhood obesity, diabetes, and eating disorders are on the increase and it is, therefore, of great concern. I appreciate that it is not always easy to overrule the pester power, but their health and well-being is really in your hands. Issues do concern them, and I think sometimes we do not give the little people the credit they are due for understanding important issues. To learn about healthy eating as a child establishes firm foundations for their future health.

Be aware of applying your own excuses to the next generation.

I taught dance and fitness for a while in a residential centre for older children with learning difficulties. The centre was based around an organic farm and they really knew their stuff. Woe betide me if I hadn't eaten what I should for tea before I met with them! They ate organic food, as far as was possible, and worked physically on the farm, and in the garden. Interestingly, this group rarely had to visit their doctor, which is highly unusual for this client group. I think there is much we can learn from this way of life.

Healthy eating is all about getting the balance right, getting into the habit of eating healthily, and arriving at the point where we no longer think, or indeed worry, about our nutrition because we know what we are eating is right and in the correct amounts. This, I believe, then frees us to focus on our spiritual walk and to get on with the work laid out before us instead of focussing so much on our selves.

How Do We Know What We Should Be Eating?

Most countries issue Government guidelines that provide information on what we should be eating, and how much, in order to maintain a healthy weight and to provide us with the required nutrients. It is worth a quick look on the internet as they provide a lot of up-to-date information and ideas. In Britain, it is the Food Standards Agency. Other useful resources are from organizations such as the local Heart, Arthritis, and Diabetic Associations' websites. These offer vast amounts of really helpful information and resources on healthy eating. You may like to order some publications for your group to share. When I run my courses, I use all their publications, order them in bulk, and send a donation to the charity. They are certainly worth a look.

There are basically five food groups that should make up a percentage of our daily food intake, but this will depend on who we are and what we are doing.

✓ Bread, rice, potatoes, pasta, and other starchy foods, around 33% of our daily intake.

✓ Fruit and vegetables, 33%

✓ Milk and dairy foods, 15%

✓ Meat, fish, eggs, beans, and other non-dairy sources of protein, 12%

X Foods and drinks high in fat and/or sugar, 7%

The first four groups are all the foods that constitute healthy eating. The last group, those foods high in fat and sugar, are not needed at all for the body to function and should, therefore, be kept to a minimum or cut out completely, which is far simpler. Let's look at each group briefly, then go into more detail about nutrients.

Group 1. Carbohydrates:

o This group contains starchy foods, such as bread, cereals, and potatoes.

o Complex carbohydrates are the best.

o This group may also include beans and lentils.

o This group **does not** contain those items that are high in sugar, such as sugary cereals. These would be included in the high fat and sugar group.

o Think of carbohydrates as ingredients in their own right.

Group 2. Fruit and Vegetables:

o Guidelines suggest at least five servings a day.

o This group is on par with the first, and we need to be looking at these two groups to make up the majority of our meals.

o Aim for a rainbow of colours.

o Fruit juice is included, but pure and not from concentrate. Beware of the sugar content.

o Frozen and tinned food is also included here. Frozen vegetables are a really useful alternative if you do not have time to prepare your vegetable. Again beware of added sugar in tinned products.

o Potatoes are not included here as they are an important carbohydrate and therefore are in the first group instead.

o Beans and lentils can also be included in this group as well as in the carbohydrate and protein groups.

Group 3. Proteins (non-dairy) - Meat, Fish, and Alternatives:

o Includes:

- Meat

- Meat products (processed)

- Eggs

- Poultry

- Fish and fish products

- Pulses, nuts, and lentils

- Beans: baked beans, butter beans, kidney beans, chickpeas, etc.

o For healthy eating, especially if you are watching your weight, it is necessary to focus on the leaner products, such as chicken and fish. Lamb, pork, and pork products, in particular, can contain high amounts of fat. Kosher is healthy!

Group 4. Milk and Dairy:

o Includes:

- Milk

- Yoghourt and milk products

- Cheese and cheese products

o This group provides a valuable source of calcium, minerals, and bacteria for a healthy digestion, but, similar to the meat group, it is important to watch the amount of fat that is in the item. Choose lower fat products where it is convenient to do so.

Group 5. Fats and Sugars:

  o It is recommended that this food group is kept to an absolute minimum. Clearly, it would be difficult to exclude all cooking oils and spreads, but low fat alternatives are best. It might be possible to exclude some items completely and to use healthier alternatives.

  o The group includes:

Unhealthy Choices		Healthier Alternatives
• All butters and margarines	→	Low fat alternatives
• Cooking oils	→	"Good oils" For example: olive oil
• Salad dressings such as mayonnaise	→	Home made or lemon juice, balsamic vinegar, olive oil, herbs
• Biscuits (cookies) and cakes	→	*Try* to keep cut down on these and have fruit instead.

  o Sugary drinks
  o Chocolate sweets crisps
  o Alcohol
  o Processed foods in general

  → Nutritionally, we do not need these. Minimal or none is good!

CARBOHYDRATES

Many people get very confused over whether we should eat carbohydrates or not. There are always arguments for and against. There is absolutely nothing wrong with including complex carbohydrates as long as you eat the correct amounts and don't serve them soaked in fat as fried bread and chips! You will also find that everyone responds differently to them and you may need to experiment a little to see exactly how you feel when you eat them. For example, I find eating too much bread leaves me feeling quite uncomfortable and sleepy, so I leave it out.

Carbohydrates are our principal source of energy. Our bodies need carbohydrates for our cells to function, and our brain runs on them! If we leave them out, it is like trying to run a car with no fuel in it. Anyone who has been on a very low calorie diet, or one that omits carbohydrates, will know not only how lethargic you become, but also how irritable and how difficult it is to concentrate. But, you may say, sugar is a carbohydrate and we are told that it is bad for you. This is not entirely true, as it is the amount consumed that causes the problem—everything in moderation. Unfortunately, we consume much greater amounts than we think due to the inclusion of "hidden" sugar in many of the products we buy. When considering which carbohydrates are better for us, we need to look at how they are structured. It is down to the make up of the carbohydrate as to which we should be eating. The majority of carbohydrates are broken down and converted into glucose (or sugar, in other words). Carbohydrates provide 4kcals/gramme. It doesn't matter where that sugar or carbohydrate comes from, it is still the same amount: Fruit sugars, milk sugars, honey, free sugars (free of a plant wall, those sugars added at the table or in cooking and manufacturing)....it is all the same. So, consider the total amounts that you are consuming. Spare fuel/energy that your body doesn't require will be stored as fat.

Carbohydrates:

- In the correct amounts, carbohydrates are the ideal fuel source for the body.

- Fats, protein, and alcohol also provide energy, but carbohydrates are the most efficient at supplying readily available energy.

There are two principal types of carbohydrates:

Carbohydrate CHO

1. Simple: Sugars
- o No nutritive value on their own
- o Exacerbates fluctuating blood sugar levels
- o Contributes to tooth decay

Examples: sucrose from cane or beet sugars, fruit sugars, milk sugars.

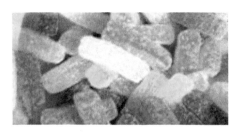

2. Complex: Starches Plus Fibre
- o The body's favourite fuel
- o Ideally should constitute 1/3 of food per day
- o Helps to avoid peaks and troughs in blood sugar
- o Energy released slower

Examples: bread, cereal, pasta, rice and beans, corn, potatoes, which also contain fibre.
KEY: Portion control

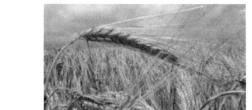

1. Simple Carbohydrates

Think: Sugar, jams, alcoholic drinks, sweets, sugary drinks, but also fruit and milk

- They are quickly broken down and absorbed into the bloodstream corresponding to a rapid rise in blood sugar levels followed by a rapid drop, frequently leaving us feeling tired.

- They are made up of very simple chains and are made of carbon, hydrogen, and oxygen.

- Most of our carbohydrates come from plants.

- If consumed in large amounts, these **simple** sugars have been found to be detrimental to our health.

- The body can manage quite well without them.

Just to make it confusing, simple sugars are also found in milk (lactose) and fruit (fructose).

So why are we encouraged to eat fruit and drink milk?

Fruit sugar is released more slowly because of the fibre that is contained in the cell wall. Milk and milk products contain valuable minerals, such as calcium, which we need for our bone health. Milk sugars and fruit sugars have been found *not* to be detrimental to our health. If you are in need of a quick pick me up, then a piece of fruit is ideal. Not only will the sugar it contains help to balance your falling blood sugar levels, but they also contain valuable nutrients and fibre.

Occasionally, simple sugars do have their uses because they can supply very quick energy….ask anyone who has run a marathon!

2. Complex Carbohydrates

Think: Oats, cereals, pasta, rice, potatoes, porridge

- The body does not break these down as quickly as the simple carbohydrates, which means they help you keep fuller for longer.

- Offer slow release energy

- These complex carbohydrates should ideally make up 1/3 of our daily food intake.

Complex carbohydrates are classified into: *Digestible* **Starch** and the *Undigestible* **Non-Starch.**

```
                          ┌─────────────────────┐
                          │    Complex CHO      │
                          └─────────────────────┘
                         ╱                       ╲
                        ╱                         ╲
   ┌──────────────────────────┐       ┌──────────────────────────────┐
   │ Digestible Starch        │       │ Undigestible Non-starch /fibre│
   │ Potatoes, cereals,       │       │ Wheat bran, celery, etc.      │
   │ beans, etc.              │       └──────────────────────────────┘
   └──────────────────────────┘                     │
                                                     ▼
                                      ┌──────────────────────────────┐
                                      │ Cellulose                    │
                                      │ (cell walls in plants)       │
                                      └──────────────────────────────┘
```

If we further consider these carbohydrates and apply this knowledge to what we are eating:

Refined versus **Unrefined**

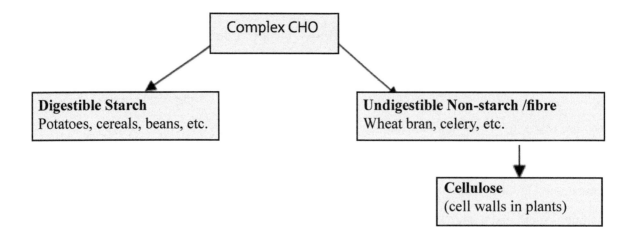

X   Refined carbohydrates - have bran and germ coats removed. Think white products, such as white

   bread. Frequently contain high levels of simple sugars.

√   Unrefined carbohydrates - contain the full grain, including the germ coat, as creation

   intended, providing us with fibre.

Why fibre?

  o   Fibre helps to slow stomach emptying and helps us to feel fuller for longer.

  o   It is essential for healthy bowel function.

  o   Fruit and vegetables contain comparable amounts of both types of fibre.

  o   Fibre may help lower cholesterol levels.

There are also two forms of fibre:

Insoluble fibre - passes through the gut mostly unchanged but absorbs water, which creates a bulkier

   stool. For example, wholegrain products such as wholegrain wheat and rye are rich in insoluble

   fibre. Bran is an insoluble fibre.

Soluble fibre - is broken down once it reaches the large bowel. For example: Oats, barley and pulses.

How much fibre?   About 18g per day is recommended, but few people eat this amount, especially if they eat a lot of processed foods and little fruit and vegetables.

Be aware:

- o If you need to increase the amount of fibre you have, do so gradually, as the gut will only adapt slowly.

- o It is also important to drink plenty of water. Most guidelines recommend 8 large glasses per day

- o People who experience such issues as Irritable Bowel Syndrome should be advised by their GP regarding fibre intake.

FATS

If carbohydrates are confusing, then fats raise the game!!

Not only are there numerous types of fat: oil, cooking oils, dipping oils, butters, and margarines, hydrogenated fats, monounsaturated fats, polyunsaturated fats, saturated fats, trans fats, to name but a few, but the information relating to them can be equally overwhelming.

So what exactly are fats? What do they do, and are they a part of healthy eating?

- o Like carbohydrates, fatty acids are made up of carbon, oxygen, and hydrogen linked together in a specific way. It is this linking that creates different molecules that make up the different fats and oils that we are familiar with on the shelves.

- o Fatty acids are split into: saturated, polyunsaturated, and monounsaturated.

- o There are fat soluble vitamins (A, D, E, and K) that need fat in the diet to be absorbed.

- o When we eat fat, the body breaks it down by hydrolysis in cells to release energy.

- o The body can utilise carbohydrates quicker, but it can also use fat.

- o Glucose from carbohydrates is easily transported around the body in the bloodstream, whereas fats are larger and need to be packaged first and then go via the digestive, lymphatic, and vascular systems.

- o The body is not very good at using fat to fuel the brain. It can, under extreme emergencies use a by-product of fat metabolism, but, if this state continues for long periods, death can result.

- o Any fat we eat that is surplus to our body's requirements is stored.

- o Fat is stored in adipose (fat) tissue.

Fat is necessary for:

❖ Insulating our bodies and our nerves.

❖ Storing and producing energy. It is our principle storage of spare energy.

❖ Helping the body to absorb the fat soluble vitamins A, D, E, and K.

❖ Transporting those fat soluble vitamins.

❖ Providing fatty acids that the body cannot produce: Essential fatty acids, such as omegas 3, 6, and 9.

❖ Promoting healthy skin and hair.

❖ Helping to regulate many physiological processes, such as maintenance of cell membranes and assistance in the regulation of the metabolism.

❖ Forming healthy plasma membranes: two fats, phospholipids and cholesterol, are important components.

❖ Providing protection for vital organs: fat surrounds and pads them.

However, we are generally eating too much fat!

As fats can be found in all of the food groups, it is important that we know what we are eating.

The Good, the Bad, and the Ugly!

There is often much confusion surrounding fats as we are encouraged to avoid this fat, eat more of that fat, this fat will make you obese, this fat will help you slim. In the end, fat is fat and we all need to eat less of it. We also need to wise up to the hidden fats present in many of the products we use, and we will look at these shortly, but first let's look at which fats we should be using. Again, the guidelines as to which we need to include are very simple. Whilst we need to keep all fats to a minimum, some types are preferential to others. Fats are similar to carbohydrates in that there are some that are better for you than others, and it is again down to their structure and origin.

"The Good"

Polyunsaturated and monounsaturated. They are exactly as their names suggest: the bonds that make these fats are unsaturated. This means that they are less stable at room temperature than the saturated fats and so exist as oils and spreads. The unsaturated fats can be beneficial to the body's functioning, including helping to alleviate inflammation and improving blood cholesterol levels, which we shall look at in more depth shortly.

Some examples of poly- and mono- unsaturated fats are:

Polyunsaturated

- Vegetable oils

- Oily fish

- Sunflower oil

- Corn oil

- Spreads made from the above

- Nuts

- Seeds

Monounsaturated

- Olive oil

- Spreads made from the above

- Hazelnuts

- Almonds

- Peanuts

- Seeds

You cannot fail to be familiar with **Omega 3, 6, and 9**, as there is so much in the media regarding these. These are all unsaturated fatty acids. Omega 3 and 6 are also known as *essential* **fatty acids** as the body cannot make them, yet they are essential for cell maintenance, including that of the brain neurons. Omega 3 and Omega 6 interact with each other so the balance between them is crucial for good health. Together they affect the production of hormonal type messengers which have an impact on inflammation in the body and all functions at a cellular level. They have also been found to help reduce mood related disorders.

Our bodies also need omega 9 fats, but we can manufacture them from other sources. Omega 9 also has many preventative qualities. Principally, Oleic acid, which you will have heard of as it is the main component of olive oil, helps to reduce the risk of atherosclerosis, cardiovascular disease, and stroke. It is, therefore, essential that they are included in what we eat. These essential fatty acids are usually found in combination with each other in foodstuffs, but examples of the principle sources are:

Omega 3	Omega 6	Omega 9
Fish oils	Eggs	Olive oil
Flaxseed	Nuts	
	Palm oil	
	Evening Primrose oil	
	Sunflower oil	

"The Bad"

Saturated fats. (*As this book goes to print, recent research is indicating that these fats may not be so "bad" as current guidelines suggest but caution in consuming too much is still advised.*) The molecules are saturated with hydrogen, which means that they are harder to break apart and have higher melting points. These bonds create the hard fats, the animal fats, including butter, lard, and cheese. It was thought that saturated fats were responsible not only for furring up the arteries, but in also raising the levels of the "bad" cholesterol in the blood. It might be wise to read up on these research developments before indulging in products full of saturated fats....moderation is always key. (As for the Hebraic perspective, the Bible in the Torah in Lev. 3:17 and 7:23 instructs us not to eat animal fat. However, fat from fowl, such as chicken and turkey is not prohibited.)

"The Ugly"

You may have heard of the terms *hydrogenated* fats and *trans* fats. These fats are effectively man made. In order to make whatever product it is more appealing, the structure of those molecules, that we mentioned earlier, that actually make up the fat, have been altered. This will produce a product that is perhaps more spreadable or that has a longer shelf life. Whilst the research continues on these fats, the evidence suggests that these fats can be quite damaging physiologically and so should be avoided. Legally, hydrogenated fats must be listed on the ingredients, but there are no regulations for trans fats at the present time. Generally, there are limited amounts in foods, BUT they can contribute to raising LDL (low density) cholesterol.

CHOLESTEROL: GOOD AND BAD

What is It and Why is There So Much Fuss About It?

Cholesterol is a fat found only animal foods, such as meat, fish, eggs, dairy. No non animal foods contain it. Cholesterol is vital to the body in many functions, including the maintenance and regulation of cells, the synthesis and creation of the sex hormones, and the production of bile acids used in digestion. Since it is essential to life, the body produces its own cholesterol from the breakdown of sugars, proteins, and fats, based on the amount of cholesterol intake in the diet.

The problem is we tend to eat too much cholesterol in animal fats. The liver then has to dispose of the excess. As mentioned, it is thought that high levels of cholesterol and possibly also saturated fats in the blood are implicated in arteriosclerosis, or the furring up of the arteries. This in turn can result in problems such as heart attacks, angina, and strokes, and it is for this reason that there is so much publicity around it.

So Why Do They Talk About "Good" Cholesterol and "Bad" Cholesterol?

As the name suggests, chole*sterol* is a sterol and is included in the lipids/fats. As such, it is more or less insoluble in water and so the body has to transport it around encapsulated in what effectively is a protein bubble, like a transporter system. These "transporters," called *lipoproteins*, come in different sizes and have different functions. The *low density lipoproteins*, LDL, are responsible for transporting cholesterol from the liver to the rest of the body. The lower the density the more fat it contains. The *high density lipoproteins*, HDL, pick up the spare cholesterol and transport it back to the liver, where it can be disposed of.

If the amount of LDL increases, it contributes to forming plaque on the walls of the arteries. This plaque eventually blocks the flow of blood with the ensuing problems, such as heart attacks and strokes. Angina is experienced when there is a partial blockage which slows the blood flow. This is why the LDL is known as the *"bad"* cholesterol. The HDL, on the other hand, actively mops up the cholesterol in order for it to be disposed of and so is referred to as *"good."*

Ways to Improve Cholesterol Levels.

The important thing to remember is that it is an overall reduction in fat consumption that will make the biggest difference. As with the carbohydrates, if you can not only cut down portion sizes but also choose healthier options, this is the key to improving your cholesterol levels. There is some evidence to suggest that substituting oleic acid (which is in olive oil) for saturated fats can help to lower LDL levels. Foods high in soluble fibre may also help to reduce cholesterol levels, such as, porridge, beans, pulses, nuts, fruits, and vegetables.

PROTEINS

- They are building blocks and are vital to life.

- They are made up of 20 different amino acids.

- Their make up is slightly more complicated than the carbohydrates and fats! These amino acids are made up of an amine group, an acid group, a hydrogen, and then also what is called an R group, which is peculiar to each particular amino acid.

- There are literally millions of different proteins, made up from these same 20 amino acids in different combinations.

- Although we often associate proteins with muscles and meat, many of them actually originate from plants. Nitrogen is taken up from the soil and this is combined with carbon from the air creating amino acids, which the plant is then able to build into proteins. Then we eat the plants directly, or the animals that have eaten the plants.

- When we eat protein, our bodies break the amino acids down and then rebuild them according to need, but, like the fatty acids, there are certain amino acids that are *essential,* that the body needs to obtain from the diet because it cannot make them itself.

We need proteins for:

Structure: Building, maintenance, and repair. Think muscles, glands, organs, cells, and connective tissue.

Balance: Homeostasis is about keeping all the cells and internal systems working in perfect balance. Think about how the body needs to control things like metabolism, blood sugar levels, fluid levels, digestion, blood clotting, and the pH balance of the blood. Specific proteins are involved in each of these processes.

Transport: As we saw in the section on cholesterol, some substances need to be transported around the body. Proteins are involved in this process, such as haemoglobin which is the protein in the red blood cells that carries oxygen around the body. If you are told you are anaemic, it means your haemoglobin levels are low, which reduces the amount of oxygen being transported.

Immune System: Besides all of the above, amino acids form antibodies to combat invading bacteria and viruses. Low levels of protein may, therefore, result in a weakened immune system.

Enzymes: Some proteins act as catalysts, that is, they speed up chemical reactions. Enzymes are needed for the breakdown of food in digestion and are involved in most cellular reactions that go on.

Energy: Proteins can also be used for energy if the sources of carbohydrate and fat are extremely low, but this system is not favoured by the body.

Whilst most western diets include sufficient protein, it is important that we eat a range of protein rich foods that will include a mixture of all the relevant amino acids. Proteins are called "complete" proteins if they contain all nine of the *essential* amino acids we spoke about, that the body cannot make for itself. These can be found in milk, meat including poultry, cheese, and eggs. The "incomplete" proteins do not have all these essential amino acids. Examples would be legumes, that is, all the beans and peas, leafy green vegetables, and the grains. As long as we are eating sufficiently, then the proteins are not something we should concern ourselves with unduly, as they do not have such a profound impact on our health as do the fats and carbohydrates. Increasing protein consumption is sometimes employed for individuals involved in heavy weight and sports training, for the repair, maintenance, and rebuilding of muscular tissue.

VITAMINS

Whilst both minerals and vitamins are required in very small amounts, measured in micro and milligrammes, they are vital to the body's functioning.

In the discussion about proteins, we mentioned enzymes that are involved in the chemical reactions within the body. Many of these enzymes require the properties of the vitamins and minerals in order to complete these tasks. There is also much evidence to suggest that eating the correct foods with the right mineral and vitamin content can have a positive impact on *mental* health.

It is not quite as clear cut as one vitamin doing one job, as many of the vitamins require another one to function properly and in some cases also require a mineral. If the balance of vitamins and minerals is not correct, their ability to work is compromised. It is not necessarily a good idea, therefore, to take a supplement of just one vitamin, unless this has been advised by someone who really knows what they are talking about. Some vitamins are stored rather than disposed of and vitamin levels can become toxic, so great care must be taken not to over consume vitamins in the mistaken belief that they are good for you and that more is better.

If you eat a well balanced diet, there should be little need for taking extra vitamin and mineral supplements, unless prescribed by your health professional. Vitamins are either fat soluble or water soluble.

Fat soluble vitamins: A, D, E and K. As the name suggests, they are found in foods that contain oil or fat. In the body they effectively "hang around" the lipids and are associated with them for their transport and storage.

Water soluble vitamins: B group and C. Because they are soluble in water, these vitamins can be easily transported by the blood system. They can also be excreted in the urine, so they do not build up so readily to toxic levels.

All vitamin levels can be reduced during food preparation, but especially the water soluble ones can be almost completely lost by over cooking.

There are endless lists available in the public domain, as to which foods are best for each vitamin, but to get you started here are a few key examples:

Vitamin	Important for:	Found in, for example:
Fat soluble:		
A	The retinoids and carotinoids. Involved in health of teeth, bone, and epithelial cells. Important for night vision. Also involved in immunity and growth.	Yellow and green vegetables. Eggs, butter, milk, fish, and fish oils.
D	Promotes calcium uptake by the small intestine and the use of phosphorus, which are required for growth, bones, teeth, and for the functioning of nerves and muscles. A good example of vitamins and minerals requiring sufficient levels of each other in order to work effectively.	Converted by sunlight. Requires approximately ½ hour in sunlight per day. Found in fish oils, eggs, and butter.
E	This vitamin is particularly important to the maintenance and smooth running of the cells, especially those of the heart and lungs. It promotes wound healing and is a powerful antioxidant.	Wholegrain cereals. palm and rice oils. liver, green leafy vegetables, some margarines.
K	Vital in the synthesis of proteins responsible for blood clotting. It is also thought to be important in the treatment of osteoporosis in increasing bone density.	Spinach, cabbage. vegetable oils, liver.

Vitamin	Important for:	Found in, for example:
Water soluble:		
C	As an antioxidant. Involved in the metabolism of proteins. Promotes health and immune function	Fruit and vegetables, especially rose-hips, oranges, and black currants. All best in their raw form.
B Group	Involved in the release of energy from food, and general metabolism. Red blood cell production.	Green vegetables, milk, liver, legumes, nuts, and intestinal bacteria.

MINERALS

The body contains about 22 minerals. Eg: Calcium, phosphorous, iron, magnesium, and zinc. Dust to dust! The majority of these, like the vitamins, are key to the body functioning correctly. They are involved in such functions as bone strength (calcium and phosphorus), energy production, muscular activity, nerve functioning (magnesium), and, as we have already discussed, production of haemoglobin, responsible for transporting oxygen around the body, which requires the mineral iron. Minerals, therefore, are vital to many physiological functions.

As a further example, many of you reading this will be familiar with the thyroid, a gland that is involved in regulating the metabolism. Iodine, in the form of iodide, is necessary for the production of the thyroid hormones. Again, similar to the vitamins, minerals react with each other and imbalances in one may compromise another. Therefore, taking just one mineral supplement can have a negative response. Minerals are taken up by plants from the soil and water, eaten by animals and then by us. A well balanced diet should supply all the necessary minerals the body requires. Refined foods, such as white bread, tend to have little mineral content.

Ten Final Points to Consider

1. Cooking Methods: They are Important

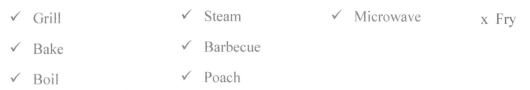

Any cooking method should ideally avoid using large amounts of fat.

2. Hidden Fats and Sugars: Watch Out For Them

Always be aware of the hidden fats and sugars that are in the products themselves or added by cooking.

Many everyday food choices can contain "hidden" amounts of fat and sugars.

Some examples are:

- o "Healthy" style flapjacks
- o Cooking sauces: cream or cheese based and pesto
- o Ready made meals
- o Coconut, as an ingredient (for example, in Asian cooking)
- o Lunch snacks
- o Take away meals
- o Battered, breaded/crumbed products
- o Cakes and biscuits (cookies)
- o Mayonnaise and salad dressings.
- o Burgers and sausages
- o Fizzy drinks and some smoothies

"Hidden" sugars may not be noticed when described by another name or foodstuff.

For example:

Brown sugar	Maltose /malt extract
Corn syrup	Maltodextrin
Dextrose	Molasses
Dried fruit	Lactose (milk sugar)
Fruit juices	Raw cane sugar
Fructose syrup	Soft brown sugar
Glucose syrup	Honey
Unrefined sugar	

How much sugar?	Contains (5g = Teaspoon)
1 can of Coca-cola	7 teaspoons
1 standard Mars bar	8.5 teaspoons
1 can of Heinz baked beans	4 teaspoons
2 fingered Kit Kat	2.5 teaspoons
1 average portion of tomato ketchup	2 teaspoons
1 can of mushy peas (a thick, lumpy pea soup)	1 teaspoons

All of these products increase the levels of fat and sugar that you will be eating. It is about cutting down on these products and making healthy substitutes rather than becoming obsessed with avoiding them at all costs. It is about wising up about the nutrition each foodstuff is providing. What is it providing for your daily needs? Is it full of vitamins and minerals, complex carbohydrate, and protein, or is the product so full of fat and sugar that your body will struggle to cope and need to store all that excess energy you are giving it as fat?

3. Salt: Consume Less

There is a substantial amount of information regarding salt and how bad it is for us, but why? Salt is made up of sodium and chloride. Sodium has been linked with high blood pressure and it is for this reason that it is suggested we have a maximum of only 1 teaspoon of salt /day. If you think of the added salt in most of the products we eat, then you can guess that most of us have far too much. I have actually trawled the supermarket to try and find products without salt, and it is extremely difficult. Similar to fat, salt enhances the flavour and we are accustomed to it. There are low sodium alternatives available, but it is better to cut down gradually. If you use a lot of salt in cooking, just try to reduce the amount you use, and it is surprising how much you can cut down without it effecting the flavour.

4. Food Labels: Read Them

Always read food labels.   Their claims of low fat and low sodium can be decieving.

Always check the amounts of these ingredients:

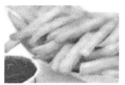 A Lot   A Little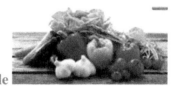

10g of added sugars	2g of added sugars
20g of fat	3g of added fat
5g of saturates	1g of saturates
1.25g of salt	0.25g of salt
.5g of sodium	0.1g of sodium
0.5g of fibre (little is bad)	3g of fibre (a lot is good)

Have a look at your Healthy Eating Checklist (on page 76) and consider if you have listed foods that:

1. Have little or no nutrient value

2. Are high in fat and sugar

3. Are high in salt

Q. How many ready-made meals or fast food portions do you have in a week? (These tend to be high in fat, sugar, and salt)

Q. How many fizzy drinks/sodas do you have in a week?

Q. How much saturated fat do you have, for example: burgers, sausages, chips, pastries, crisps, burgers, cakes, and biscuits?

5. Antioxidants: What Are They and Do I Need Them?

In the normal every day functioning of the body a process called oxidation takes place. By-products of this process are called free radicals. These free radicals are extremely unstable and can damage other cells if left to their own devices. Antioxidants, as their name implies, can neutralize these free radicals. In brief, we need to eat plenty and a wide variety of fruits and vegetables.

6. Blood Sugar Levels: Control Them

For anyone who is diabetic, they will know only too well that we need to keep our blood sugar levels as stable as possible. For the rest of us, it is not something that we usually think about, or even understand. Greatly fluctuating blood sugar levels have a great impact on how the body responds and it can be fatal!

We mentioned earlier that if we eat high levels of simple carbohydrates, the body absorbs these quickly into the blood stream and blood sugar levels rise dramatically. If this is not used immediately by physical activity, it is then followed by a sharp fall and we will feel tired and lethargic. The reason for this drop in blood sugar level is because as levels of sugar in our blood rise, the hormone insulin is released that helps to control it. As we consume large amounts of sugar, the insulin will compensate and will bring blood sugar levels down by encouraging the body to absorb it and store it. The blood sugar is effectively taken out of circulation, which leaves us tired and lethargic. If we continue to feed ourselves high levels of sugar then our bodies can become less effective at controlling it.

Regulating blood sugar is important, and if we aim to keep it stable, it helps us to have a steady supply of energy throughout the day. What we eat and how often helps to regulate this.

Have a look at the two blood sugar level examples on the next page and answer the following questions referring to your Healthy Eating Checklist (on page 76).

Q. What would your blood sugar levels look like?

Q. What kind of meals do you eat? Are they well planned and nutritionally balanced?

Q. What kinds and sizes of snacks do you eat?

Q. Look again at the blood sugar illustrations on the next page and choose which one is closer to the way you eat. Would your day be more like the red or the blue?

Example 1

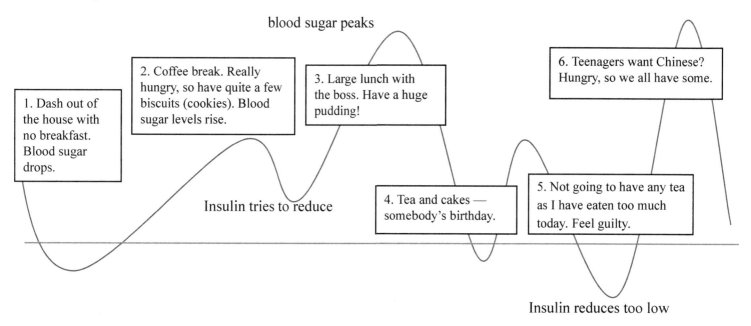

Constant Blood Sugar Level

Greatly fluctuating blood sugar

Example 2

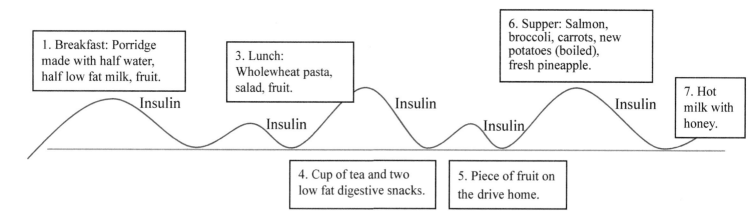

Constant Blood Sugar

Gently fluctuating blood sugar levels

You can see from these two examples the difference in blood sugar levels. Ideally, of course, you are aiming for the second example. This is really all about planning. If you are feeling a bit low and in need of a snack, a piece of fruit is an ideal way to boost your blood sugar levels safely. As we have already discussed, try to base your meals around complex carbohydrates, fruits, and vegetables. If you eat regular meals containing the right, nutritionally balanced foodstuffs, there is no reason to feel hungry or to run out of energy.

7. Glycemic Index Values: What Are They and Should I Be Considering Them?

Glycemic index (GI) is a method that is used to measure what effect a particular food product has on blood sugar levels. So, if you consider both the two examples we have just looked at, and also the food groups that should be making up the bulk of our meals, different foodstuffs can be used to regulate our blood sugar. Those with a high GI value will give you a sudden rush of blood sugar, whereas those foods with a low or medium GI value will provide a slow release of energy. Just to confuse the issue, it is not necessarily as we expect, and so it is helpful to be familiar with what foodstuffs are high, medium, and low. For example, it also depends on what else you eat the food with and how the food is prepared. There are a number of books available that catalogue the index of most foods and also, of course, you can look online. Here is a quick summary list:

- Foods with a high GI- soft drinks, bread, and honey.
- Foods with a moderate GI - porridge, pasta, grapes.
- Foods with a low GI – apples, milk, yoghourt, grapefruit.

A number of diet programmes, currently on the market, are based around the GI. Whilst these programmes are quite usable, they are, at the end of the day, another form of a diet, and I would like to think that you can move away from having to focus so intently on what you eat all the time. My hope is that once you get into eating more healthily, you will know what you can and can't include, and you will no longer have to think so much about food. Cut Loose!!

8. Super Foods: Do They Exist?

The market is extremely good at convincing us that we "need" certain items. Superfoods, as they are called, may contain high amounts of a certain mineral or vitamin, or antioxidant, but no food is the "miracle" cure all. No one food is going to make us thin overnight or cure our aches and remove all our wrinkles. THE only way towards improved health is eating a healthy, balanced diet and to exercise......so don't waste your money.

9. Portions: How Much Should I Be Eating?

We will look at portion sizes when we consider long term weight loss, but suffice to say at this juncture that most of us eat far too much. It is important to be aware of our physical hunger and to eat when we are physically hungry, which is the next point.

10. Hunger: How and Why Do I Get Hungry?

There are many types of hunger that the specialists can identify, but these are the basic three:

- ❖ **Real physiological hunger:** You are familiar with a rumbling stomach and a headache or feeling a little light headed. This is the hunger we need to focus on.
- ❖ **Sensory hunger:** You know what this is like. It's when your mouth starts to water with the smell, sight, and taste as well as the memory of a particular food.
- ❖ **Emotional hunger:** This is when we eat because of our emotions, such as anxiety, stress, anger, and boredom. This results in comfort eating or sometimes not eating at all. It is this psychology of eating that is involved with eating disorders.

The graphic on the next page illustrates two more types of hunger:

- ❖ **Habitual hunger:** This is when we eat just because it's the time to eat according to what we've done all our lives or according to tradition, etc.
- ❖ **Social hunger:** You have overnight guests and must feed them the traditional meals and snacks, or you are invited for a meal or coffee, or to a wedding, etc. Of course you eat what is served and when it is served.

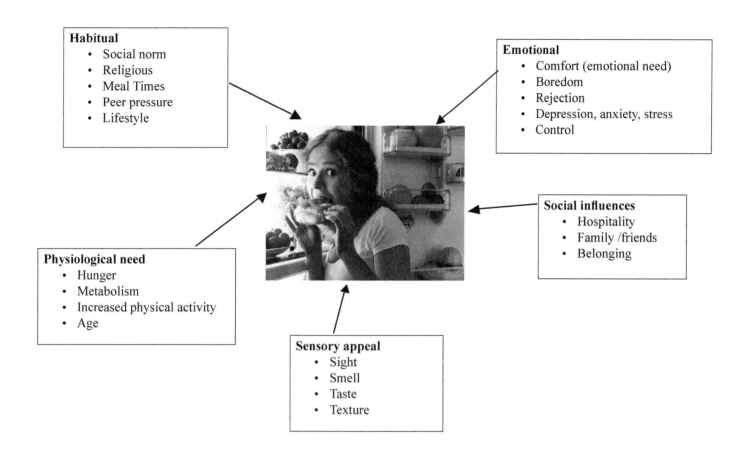

Habitual
- Social norm
- Religious
- Meal Times
- Peer pressure
- Lifestyle

Emotional
- Comfort (emotional need)
- Boredom
- Rejection
- Depression, anxiety, stress
- Control

Physiological need
- Hunger
- Metabolism
- Increased physical activity
- Age

Social influences
- Hospitality
- Family /friends
- Belonging

Sensory appeal
- Sight
- Smell
- Taste
- Texture

Physiologically, there are two important hormones that regulate hunger, ghrelin and leptin. Ghrelin is responsible for a desire to eat and leptin tells us that we have had sufficient. If we consider these in conjunction with a healthy eating programme, ideally, we need to eat foods that will activate the hormone leptin. These include any healthy foods such as fruits, nuts, vegetables and lean meats. Lack of sleep has also been found to be associated with low levels of Leptin. Difficulty with sleeping is a common disturbance with people who are significantly overweight and obese, which further exacerbates overeating and hunger control. If we continuously overeat, our sensitivity to leptin is reduced and we can no longer tell if we are full.

Menopause

You are probably wondering why on earth I am mentioning the menopause here? The answer lies in the fact that many of the symptoms women experience pre, during, and post menopause can be influenced by what they eat. If you experience such issues as:

- Mood swings
- Hot flushes
- Aging skin
- Joint pains
- Weight gain (over and above normal fluctuations)
- Headaches
- Night sweats

Then you are probably cruising somewhere in menopause (personal experience!). There are some excellent resources on dealing with the menopause naturally and it is worth looking around a bit to see what suits you best.

Summary of Healthy Eating Points

Carbohydrates

- Lower in calories than fatty foods: **1g = 4 calories**

- Try and make your meals based around complex starchy carbohydrates. They will help to keep you fuller for longer and provide valuable fibre. Eg. Potatoes, pasta, rice, and cereals.

- Wherever possible, aim for wholegrain varieties.

- Try and keep sugary items to a minimum, especially drinks.

- Be aware of "hidden" sugars. Read the labels.

- Try and cut down on sugar in hot drinks—try half teaspoon less each time.

- Try and avoid "malted grains" as malt is a simple sugar.

- Be aware of how you cook your complex carbohydrates:
  Try to stick to boiling, steaming, baking, and mashing.
  Avoid frying.
  Avoid making creamy sauces. Try tomato based ones instead.

Alternative healthier choices:

Frosted cereals   →   Whole grain cereals

White toast   →   Wholemeal toast

White pasta   →   Wholemeal pasta

White rice   →   Brown /wild rice

KEEP IT SIMPLE, FRESH, and WHOLESOME.
AVOID PROCESSED FOODS where possible.

Fats

o The most concentrated form of energy: **1g = 9 calories.**

o Try and keep fats to a minimum, but don't leave it out altogether.

o Aim to use the "good" fats for cooking and baking: mono and polyunsaturated.

o Try to avoid using too much fat in food preparation, such as in frying.

o Stick to low fat alternatives. Check the labels: sometimes low fat means high sugar.

o Try and use lean cuts of meat and skinless chicken.

Protein

o Also lower in calories than fat: **1g = 4 calories**

o Try and stick to the leaner cuts of meat to avoid high fat intake.

o Eat a mix of protein to ensure you get all the right amino acids.

Fruit and Vegetables

o Low in calories, high in fibre, great at filling you up.

o Rich in vitamins and minerals and come in their own packaging.

o Help to build a robust immune system.

o If you do not particularly like fruit, or object to the preparation time, make a fruit salad and keep it in the fridge. Grapes are a good item to have around to nibble on.

o Likewise, if you or your family are not keen on vegetables, use them in soups and stews. Beans and lentils are excellent at bulking meals out cheaply.

o Frozen vegetables and fruit without added sugar are a good alternative, especially if you are in a hurry.

Sugary Foods

o Sugary foods are high in calories with little or no nutritive value.

o If a product advertises that it is low in sugar, it is often high in fat and vice versa.

o Alcohol is simply sugar in a glass.

Moderation ….cut down ….cut out ….cut loose ….your body doesn't need it.

Is not Creation simply amazing in its intricate design?

These complex mechanisms that you have read about in this chapter make up your physical body—that clay jar —the Temple of the Holy Spirit—designed perfectly.

"I thank you because I am awesomely made, wonderfully; your works are wonders

—I know this very well."

Psalm 139:14

Chapter Six – Mood, Food, and Other Hurdles

Introduction

In this chapter, I would like to look briefly at some of the issues that can have a significant impact on our quality of life, such as comfort eating, body image, self-esteem, and confidence.

Q. If we are to be "living sacrifices" and to have our focus on Yahweh, then why is there so much emphasis on "self" esteem today?

These concerns are connected with how we think, our feelings and emotions, and how we view ourselves. So, I would like to continue to apply what we considered in Part One and to look at these issues through our Biblical spectacles. Let's consider the renewing of our minds and focusing on who we are in Him.

Again, I am no specialist, but I do work in the field of mental ill health and personally went through many years of what is now officially termed binge eating disorder, and so I write this chapter with both professional and personal experience. I am hoping that some of it may be helpful to you in both recognising these difficulties and also in giving you, at least a few, down to earth practical suggestions. Please remember that I am simply writing down my own experiences and that which I firmly believe Yeshua has taught me along the way. You need to continue to test and approve these words and to act accordingly.

I am going to take time out here and use my own personal experiences to explain how these emotional cycles can so easily ensnare us and how God can and does completely heal us. Perhaps some of you reading this will find it all too familiar.

As a teenager, and into my twenties, I went through what was an emotional roller coaster. I had an extremely happy childhood and a wonderful supportive family. I had no obvious reason to slide into the situation I was finding myself in, but as I went through my teenage years when needing to find my own identity, I experienced extremely low moods. I now know that much of it probably had to do more with hormones than mental health, but in this respect hindsight is not that helpful.

When it all started, I was extremely active and busy. I was at sixth form college (grades 12 and 13) and working at the local riding school as often as I could, walking the 4 miles there and then back in the evening after a full day of yard work and horse back riding. I also sailed dinghies and enjoyed mountain walking and going off camping and travelling. I was in all the high school games teams and even went for the county basketball trials. Despite all this activity, I remained very overweight, reaching 14 stone (196 pounds) at one stage.

I was lost and had no understanding of how to lose weight safely. I would starve myself for days at a time, lying to my parents and telling them I had eaten at school. This would then lead to a binge cycle where I would sneak into the kitchen at night and just eat anything I could find. I would also buy vast amounts of food and eat it in secret, usually high fat sugary items that I didn't even particularly like. I became an expert at hiding any evidence.

It was like being in a trance-like state where I would not register the reality of what I was doing. The guilt and self-loathing that would follow these binges was insurmountable. I hated myself so much that I would hit myself until I bruised. I would stand in front of the mirror crying and telling myself how much I hated myself and how I thought of myself as a parasite. To the outside world, of course, everything was just hunky dory.

Early on, I became friendly with a lovely Christian girl, Pamela, whilst we were still in the sixth form. I had always been to church with my family but had never really thought about faith or what I believed in. This lovely lady invited me to her church, a little church in the middle of a waste building sight in the town where we lived. The Pastor there at the time was a vibrant Welsh man who gave fiery sermons that were enough to challenge any rebellious teenager. It was there, on 25th January 1976, that I gave my heart, finally, to Yeshua, and it was there that the healing began, that still continues today.

It took me many years to learn how to manage my emotions and to bring them all to Yahweh. I took two years off of studying after leaving the 6th form and then went on to attend Agricultural College. Throughout all these years, there was a continuous battle with my eating and an endless round of diets, even though I now knew Yeshua as my personal Saviour. I was, and still am, extremely independent, always thinking I can do it all myself. Slowly but surely, though, Yahweh put people in my path that headed me in the right direction, taught me about eating more healthily, and encouraged me to accept myself as who I am in Yeshua.

I still experience feelings and emotions that rear their ugly heads every so often, and I can still lapse into a need for comfort food. The big *however,* though, is that I am now in control through His strength. This is the complete workable healing He has given me. It wasn't overnight or miraculous in any way, but a long slow learning experience. It keeps me on my toes and is a constant reminder of His love for me. I accept who I am in Yeshua HaMashiach (the Messiah) and not who the world demands that I be. This is a pretty cool place to be and I hope you are there with me. Trust completely. Ask and He *will* heal you…..freedom indeed!

Back to Basics

If you think back to the studies in Part One, we looked more closely at our being spirit, soul, and body. We considered the soul as being that of our "world consciousness," our "psychy," of the mind, our decision-making process. So think now of what is the basis for the issues we are considering here. It might be helpful if you also take another look at the diagrammes towards the end of Study 5, through which we aimed to establish where we looked to for our direction, the world, or Yahweh?

If we simply take on board what the world is telling us and we are not emotionally robust, then we are likely to become entangled in all the issues we are discussing here as a means of coping with our emotional needs. If we look to our Heavenly Father, however, then that is where we find our security, our **firm foundations,** and our every confidence in who we are in Him.

"Moreover, my God will fill every need of yours according to his glorious wealth, in union with the Messiah Yeshua."

Philippians 4:19

If you would, continue to apply these principles as we now consider briefly a few of these issues. We need to consider these areas before looking at weight management, as they can and will act as substantial barriers to achieving a healthy approach to food if we are not aware of what is happening and where they originate.

Comfort Eating and Disordered Eating

Is There a Connection Between Mood and Food?

I would confidently state that the majority of the people I see professionally have what can be described as disordered eating, that is, as the name describes. I consider it as an unhealthy way of eating, skipped meals, overeating, frequently dieting, constantly thinking about what you can and cannot eat, and a distorted approach to food in general. I would also place issues such as yo-yo dieting in this category, which we will look at in the next chapter, only because it is, in some instances, exacerbated by emotional responses. These matters are rarely recognised for what they are as so many people experience the same, and they easily become habitual and the norm.

I am going to speak in general terms here as the intricacies of eating disorders are not my field. If the way you are eating, or not eating as the case may be, is damaging your health, physically and mentally, then an eating disorder may well be diagnosed. These include the conditions of anorexia, bulimia nervosa, and binge eating. If you know that you, or your loved ones, are experiencing any of these, then it is **imperative** that you seek help.

I am going to stick my head above the parapet and say that I consider that both comfort eating and disordered eating are one step away from these diagnosable illnesses. For this section, I am not merely talking of having a few too many cookies, or an occasional cream cake. Rather, a way of eating that is driven by your emotions and feelings and one that impacts on your way of thinking and your physical and mental well-being in general. It is not the food consumed that is the problem, but why we are eating it in the first place. Eating is simply the tiny tip of an enormous iceberg of emotional need. These patterns of eating are triggered by an inability to both recognise, and deal with, our emotions. It can also be a method of control and for some, a way of dealing with extremely painful situations or trauma. It can be self-generating, with feelings of guilt and a sense of failure creating an environment that results in bingeing cycles, or starvation. Emotional eating is a coping strategy and in that sense is the same as some people use alcohol or drugs. It is a method of soothing ourselves because we know of no other way, having never learned how to manage our feelings. Emotional eaters don't wait to feel hungry and often are not aware of the body's signals, neither will they feel comfortably satisfied as you would after a pleasant meal, and I speak from personal experience

Overcoming Emotional Eating

First and foremost, spiritually, I suggest that these issues must be prayed through with someone, bringing them to the foot of the Cross and then leaving them there. Ask that Yahweh would guide, direct, strengthen, and support you as you seek to deal with these hurdles. Continue to support each other and don't be afraid of being firm as well as positive. Frequently I have to be quite assertive in getting my clients to see that this depends on their own choice to act. (Re-read the cycle of change if necessary in Chapter 2.) I am not by any means diminishing the task ahead as it can appear quite overwhelming, but it is also extremely easy to give up and use our weaknesses to hide behind. Sometimes this chaotic way of eating stems from traumatic events that may have happened years ago. If you need extra outside professional help, ASK. Fortunately, I had the right people in the right place to help push me forward to actually do something for myself and to support me. Your Heavenly Father does not want you in this state and the enemy will use your weaknesses if you give him this open door.

Stop Striving and Allow God to Work

To be practical, there is much you can do, with Yahweh's help that is pro-active. Here are just a few suggestions:

1. **Identify Your Triggers**

> Why are you comfort eating?
>
> Why are you not eating?

I encourage my own clients to keep a Truth diary. Jot down why, when, and where you resort to eating, or when, where, and why you just stop eating. If you are honest with yourself, you may well see a pattern emerging that you hadn't even considered. You don't have to keep these for long before you will see where things are going peculiar.

Common Triggers:

Rejection	Loneliness
Anger / frustration	Worries –financial, work, housing
Stress/fatigue	Relationship difficulties
Depression / anxiety	Boredom / habit
Health problems	Unemployment
Exams / assessments	Overwhelmed
Sadness	Fear

2. **Deal With the Triggers**

As we have just discussed, without dealing with the emotions that are driving you to eat, you won't be able to move on. So, once you have identified the problem, bring it to Adonai in prayer. Try and find practical solutions, and if you need help or advice, ask for it.

3. Explore the Alternatives

Discover alternative coping mechanisms and learn to be kind to yourself. If at this point you dislike yourself, as I did, or you are fiercely independent, the bread winner, the one that doesn't need help, then being kind to yourself is not something you will be very good at. BUT, take it from me, the harder you try, the easier it becomes. So instead of heading to the nearest fast food shop, learn to use alternative ways of dealing with the emotional turmoil.

Take a minute out to yourself before reaching for the cookie jar; breathe deeply; think about what is causing you concern. Have you addressed it already? If so, deny those little voices any ground, if not, then write them in your truth diary and consider how you can manage them optimally.

You may need more than one alternative, so make a list of ideas and activities that are suited to each situation when you find yourself craving the fat and sugar.

- ❖ Pray and ask someone to pray with you. When two or three are gathered together....
- ❖ BELIEVE He loves you enough to answer your prayers!!
- ❖ Read Scripture that uplifts you.
- ❖ Speak to someone, phone a friend. (Rely on your support network.)
- ❖ Walk the dog.
- ❖ Visit friends.
- ❖ Get lost in a good book.
- ❖ Have a bubble bath.
- ❖ Dig the garden.
- ❖ Take a break, just five minutes of deep breathing can help if you are office bound.

There is now a plethora of evidence that shows that **physical activity** is good for lifting your mood. So, get out in the fresh air, walking, cycling, gardening, or simply wandering. Any physical activity is better than not doing anything, so it really doesn't matter what you do as long as you enjoy it. If it is a good positive experience, then you will soon register that it can be just as good as comforting yourself with food. Look after yourself, eat healthily and plan meals carefully, get sufficient sleep, and take time to have space for yourself, even if it is just a few minutes where you simply stop.

4. Find Support

A good support network makes life so much easier. If no one immediately comes to mind, it may be helpful to join a local support group.

5. Identify Physical vs Emotional Hunger

Learn to identify when you are physically hungry. Learn the signals that your body is giving you, rather than your head and your heart. Try and be self aware.

6. Slow it Down

It takes a little while for the body to register that it is feeling full and to relay the signals to your brain, in fact about twenty minutes, so eat slowly and allow yourself to enjoy your meal. Set the table and take your time, even if you are just you. I often eat whilst I'm reading the paper if I'm on my own which works really well.

7. Strategically Plan Your Shopping

It is not a good idea to shop if you are really feeling emotionally vulnerable, unless it is absolutely necessary. The best time is after a meal, when you are full and comfortable. It is also a good idea to make a shopping list before you see the food, and then stick to it! If you really don't need the food that you normally comfort eat, then don't buy it.

8. Avoid Mindless Snacking

If you are trying to overcome emotional eating, then don't trip yourself up by taking unplanned snacks. Try and be more conscious of what you put in your mouth. Prepare healthy snacks in advance.

Low Self-Esteem, Lacking in Confidence, Poor Body Image

How often do we see advice on boosting self-esteem and building self-confidence or how to improve your body image? You can even do courses in it. I am also guilty of using it on my advertising in the past. You see it everywhere and it is what people are looking for. The media is overloaded with celebrities losing it, having buckets of it, talking about it, teaching about it, so what is **it**?

Have a look at the dictionary definitions of the following:

Self-esteem:

Confidence:

Confident:

Self-confidence:

> If you have it available, have a glance back at the "Quick Quiz" you completed in Bible Study 4 on pages 32-35. Reflect on what you wrote regarding how you see yourself.

If we summarise the above, they are all concerned with how I view myself, what I think of myself, and how I evaluate what I am capable of. In studying this further, I believe we can identify two very different conclusions. The first is that we have a basic natural opinion of ourself that knows who we are and what we are capable of. The second is that our self-esteem and confidence can create in us a sense of superiority, pride, and arrogance or, at the opposite end of the scale, a sense of self-loathing—all of which focuses on self. If you look at the definitions for self-esteem above, you will see a fairly clear distinction between the two.

As a further example, I have a great friend who was good enough to go to the Olympics for the windsurfing event. She also ran for a well-known athletics club and could have competed in top events if she had so chosen. If you didn't know her, you would think she was extremely arrogant about her sporting ability, but anyone who really knows her, sees that she is a very unassuming and shy individual and soon realises that she simply knows what she is capable of. This I believe is the subtle difference.

Keep the Biblical Perspective

If you think back to Bible Study 3 in the "Chasing Rainbows" section, we looked at how the world is driven to please the self and indeed how the world dictates who we are and what we should look like. We looked at the larger picture and considered subjects such as hedonism, humanism, and narcissism, which are ultimately all to do with pleasure, the ability of man to manage without God, and the pleasing of self. You may ask, what has this got to do with me feeling good about myself? Well, I am going to suggest that we need our opinion of our self and its capabilities to be who we are as centred and grounded in Yahweh.

This might be stating the obvious, but just as comfort eating can so easily become a habit, I believe so can a worldly opinion of ourself. It is about constantly maintaining a spiritual perspective. In effect it has to be "*who we are in Yeshua esteem*" and to have our confidence in what we are capable of, completely grounded in Him. There is simply nothing within me that is of any use or any good. Any good that is in me comes from that which my Heavenly Father has equipped me with. Therefore, my self-esteem, confidences, and the thoughts I have of my own physical body, need to reflect the work that He has done in me and not who I am as self, because that "ain't no pretty sight."

1 John 2:16-17

"Because all the things of the world—the desires of the old nature, the desires of the eyes, and the pretensions of life—are not from the Father but from the world."

Phillipians 4:13 "I can do everything through him who gives me power."

And of course He will set us far higher tasks than we ever think we are capable of!

If we keep this Biblical perspective, it can have a huge impact on the changes we make and our attempts to maintain a healthier lifestyle.

Before we finish this chapter, I would like to consider two further points. The first is that there are many individuals who have a genuinely low opinion of themselves and this, in its extreme, can be debilitating.

By way of example, I had one lady that attended my classes who was quite beautiful, had three fabulous sons and a caring and loving husband. To all intents and purposes, you would imagine this lady to be confident and to have a positive opinion of herself. However, the reality was quite different. From an early age, she had attended a horrendous boarding school. The treatment of the children at this school would hit the headlines if it existed today. Not only this, but also the sense of not being wanted at home, as a child, was overwhelming for her. This was not actually the case, it was simply that her mother was too busy to adequately care for her

24/7, but as a child, she was unable to interpret the facts from how she felt. As a result, this wonderful lady had a genuine extremely low opinion of herself. In fact, it was as if she had absolutely no opinion of herself. It was as if it was too painful to consider who she was. She was also an incredible artist, but because her sister was an artist by profession, she would brush aside all attempts at praising her for her art by saying things like, "You should see my sister's paintings. Mine are nothing in comparison." For this lady, any form of compliment would run off like water down a greasy pole. The only way her friends could help was to constantly encourage her so that eventually a little confidence crept in.

The way we behave and react to circumstances and what people say is directly influenced by the way we feel, which in turn is both controlled and maintained by the thoughts in our heads. The way we think is established and influenced by our experiences. We effectively learn through these experiences. Significant situations that we experience, especially with regard to our beliefs about our self, in time, shape our feelings and our subsequent behaviours and reactions, either negatively or positively. These include our experiences in childhood, adolescence, and as adults, just like the lady I have just described.

If you constantly use phrases such as: "I always make a mess of things"; "I am such a waste of space"; "I am so ugly"; "There's no point in trying" then you are constantly reinforcing your own negative thinking. These negative thought patterns can also be maintained by errors in our all or nothing thinking, such as, "Unless I am the best, I am a complete failure," and jumping to conclusions and saying things like, "They don't like me," and "I'm bound to fail."

BUT, what does all this say about how we were created and how valuable we are to Yahweh?

Re-read Psalm 139

The good news is that this way of thinking, which can be quite destructive, can be addressed.

Focus on and remember that:

> "You were bought at a price, do not become slaves of men"
> **1 Corinthians 7:23**

This is the value that God puts on you, that He sent His own Son to the cross for you. Be careful, therefore, not to diminish what He has done by telling yourself you are not worth it. Neither be condemned by your thinking, rather pray for healing and the wherewithal to change.

We have already looked at behavioral change, and the way to overcome this negative thinking is much the same. It is also similar, in that it is your choice and only you can activate the change in your thinking.

Try the Following

Stop Criticizing Yourself!

Everyone at some point or other, gets those little voices that tell them they are no good, that they are too fat, too tall—all those words of accusation. It helps if you can get to the point where you actively choose not to indulge in this constant self-criticism. Without really thinking about it, negative thoughts pop into our heads completely unchallenged and can become self fulfilling prophecies. Next time this happens, just stop yourself and think about what you are telling yourself. At the risk of sounding flippant, at these times, I just do what children do best. I say, "I can't hear you!" (You don't have to necessarily do the bit where you also run off into the garden whilst putting your hands over your ears, unless you really feel this helps!)

Acknowledge Your Achievements!

Focus on how you can change your thinking to embrace a positive mindset.   There are a number of things you can do to help yourself. All of them will go a long way to building your self-worth in Yahweh.

o   List your achievements and congratulate yourself.

o   Learn to be kind to yourself.

o   The negative thoughts are *not* facts! Read Scripture to find the truth!!

o   Make a list of Bible verses that contradict your negative thoughts.

o   Read those verses aloud to yourself several times a day.

o   Avoid **"should" and "must"** statements.

o   If something goes wrong, in whatever context, forgive yourself and move on.

o   Encourage and treat yourself.

o   Learn a new skill/hobby. Mastery of something new really helps.

o   Do something amazing for charity.

Get Professional Help!

Of great importance, if you, or someone you know, has a genuine struggle with these issues then I suggest, again, that you seek further help. Body Dysmorphic Disorder is connected to our body image. It is about having a distorted image of your own body and generally involves viewing one body part as being unacceptable to the point of hatred. This is a mental health problem and is far more common than you would expect. It is just as destructive as any of the eating disorders and, again, it is imperative that help is sought. If you find it too intimidating asking your own doctor, look for a national organisation that specialises in these areas.

Watch Out for Pride and False Humility!

Proverbs 16:18-19

"Pride goes before destruction, and arrogance before failure. Better to be humble among the poor than share the spoil with the proud."

Whilst this following passage is discussing the future of Edom, there is a healthy message here about getting the balance correct and how easily we can be deceived.

Jeremiah 49:16 "'Your capacity to terrorize has deceived you and made you arrogant. You make your home in the rocky crags and seize the top of the mountain; but even if you build your nest high as an eagle's, from there I will drag you down,' says ADONAI."

The opposite of pride is, of course, humility. We are encouraged to remain humble and we are warned against pride, but we can sometimes overdo the theatrics and bounce to the other end of the scale. We need to be aware of this as it creeps in when we are not expecting it. I think we are all guilty of displaying it at some time or another. This is a tricky one as the world has made it very trendy to state "I lack confidence" or "I dislike myself so much" as a way of being the centre of attention. What these statements are actually saying are, "Can you please reassure me that I am acceptable to you." So, beware of a humility that results in an opting out of responsibility.

And Finally

If these issues are affecting you or any of your loved ones significantly, it is **vital** that you seek further professional help. I fully appreciate that it is not easy asking for help, and that denial is a powerful agent. Men especially have a hard time with these issues, as it is extremely difficult for men to admit they need help. **BUT,** I do ask that, after reading this, if necessary, you get in touch with a suitable professional or elder. Yes, this can be an extremely painful process to go through, but you don't have to go it alone and it is about cutting the chains that bind. Your Heavenly Father offers you freedom and freedom indeed! Cut loose!

Please read:

Psalm 142:6-7 (NIV)

"Listen to my cry, for I am in desperate need; rescue me from those who pursue me, for they are too strong for me. Set me free from prison that I may praise your name"

Luke 4:18-19 (NIV) (from Isaiah 61)

" The Spirit of the Lord is on me, because he has anointed me to preach good news to the poor. He has sent me to proclaim freedom for the prisoners and recovery of sight for the blind, to release the oppressed, to proclaim the year of the Lord's favour "

Re-read John 10:10 (NIV)

"The thief comes only to steal and kill and destroy; I have come that they may have life, and have it to the full."

And for further encouragement, read Psalm 61.

Chapter Seven – Weight Management – Long Term

Introduction

We have just looked at the foundations you need for eating more healthily. This chapter is about how to embrace eating healthily in terms of weight management. We will be looking primarily at long term healthy weight loss. This is very different from putting yourself on a diet for reasons I will explain shortly. This is about eating healthily and happily for the rest of your life, enjoying your food and eating for vitality. It is also about being comfortable with what you are eating, being free from the emotional roller coasters of yesterday, and cutting loose from the dictates of the world as to what size and shape you should be.

We will also look at weight gain. Whilst people who need to increase their weight are generally in the minority, it is by far the harder of the two to achieve. This chapter is all about taking a safe and effective approach to weight management that is not only going to last, but that is also healthier for yourself and honouring to your Heavenly Father.

What is a Healthy Weight?

THE most important point here is that we are considering not total body weight, but body composition. I cannot stress this enough because just getting on the scales everyday is not going to tell you what you need to know (throw them away!). It is about your **fat to lean ratio.** In terms of measuring body composition, your body can be divided into fat or adipose tissue and lean tissue, which is all the rest, your bones and organs, muscles and tissues. As an example, take two individuals who are an identical weight:

Person 1	**Person 2**
Male 22	Male 22
Competitive athlete	IT consultant
Weight: 12 stone (168 lbs.)	12 stone (168 lbs.)
Height: 6 ft.	6 ft.
Body Fat: 18%	35%

So, when these two individuals get on the weighing scales, they weigh the same. The difference is the amount of fat they are carrying, which is clearly quite different.

The principal issue usually is the amount of visceral fat around the abdomen, that is, the "unhealthy" fat that is laid down around your internal organs. This is particularly important for men who sport the rather large tummy, which is an indicator of risk for heart and metabolic complications. Whereas some store fat around their middle, most men tend to store it around the organs, which is especially dangerous.

Much research is still being carried out as to the best way to measure how fat we are and the amount that each individual needs to lose. Currently two methods are widely utilised, **Waist Measurement** and **Body Mass Index (BMI)**. These are used as helpful guides in establishing the level at which we are over or under weight. These two measurements provide a good baseline from which to work and also prevent you from being plunged into depression every time you step on the scales.

Waist Measurement

By using waist measurement, we can gauge the amount of visceral fat someone has. Having high deposits of this visceral fat is considered an important indicator of risk for many of the weight associated illnesses: metabolic disorders like diabetes and heart problems, such as coronary heart disease (CHD). The following table shows those categories that equate to an increased risk of health complications.

	Waist	
Men	> 94cm (37 in.)	Increased risk of CHD
Men	> 102 cm (40 in.)	Severely increased risk of CHD
Asian Men	> 90 cm (35.5 in.)	Increased risk of CHD
Women	> 80 cm (31.5 in.)	Increased risk of CHD
Women	> 88 cm (34.6 in.)	Severely increased risk of CHD

Body Mass Index (BMI).

You may well have been told your BMI by your GP, but it is quite easy to work it out for yourself. BMI is a measure of your body mass in relation to your height. However, again, it can only be used as a guide as it does not distinguish between body fat and lean tissue.

BMI is calculated by dividing weight (Kg) by the square of the height (metres).

For example, someone weighing 75kg (165 lbs.) who is 1.75 m (5'9") in height:

$$BMI = \frac{75}{(1.75 \times 1.75)} = \frac{75}{3.06} = 24.5$$

Guidelines for healthy BMI are as follows:

BMI Ranges:	
Underweight	<18.5
Normal Range	18.6-24.9
Overweight	25- 29.9
Obese Class 1	30-34.9
Obese Class 2	35-39.9
Obese Class 3	>40
Super morbid obese	>50
End stage obesity syndrome	>60

Both of these above methods are easy to use and, used together, are a helpful guide to help you keep tabs with how well you are doing when trying to lose/gain weight.

The majority of people are well aware and know if they need to consider weight loss, or weight gain, but identifying what weight you need to be ideally is something a little less tangible. For our purposes, it is about what is a healthy weight for you as an individual and not what society dictates that you be. If my clients ask me what weight they "should" be, I always ask them what weight they think. They generally expect me to come up with an exact figure, but I have found that it is better to have a more practical approach. Gaining weight for those who need to is very hard, and therefore most of them are only too pleased to be any weight as long as it is slightly heavier than they were. For weight loss, I suggest that you will find a weight that you are comfortable with, that you feel healthy at, and that you are able to maintain reasonably easily. We will look at maintenance shortly, but you will find that this is the weight at which your body will "sit" nicely. Much of this comes down to your genetics and your body type. Sometimes these skip a generation, so you may look more like your grandparents, but you will look like someone in your family in terms of body shape and size.

Body Type: Which One Are You?

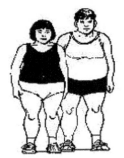

Endomorph

We are often a bit of a mixture.

Endomorph
Features: wider hips than shoulders, small bones, generally round in shape, gains weight easily.

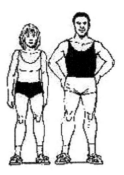

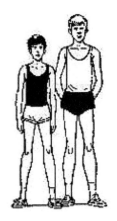

Ectomorph
Features: equal hips to shoulders, long, slim, boyish, low body fat, low potential for muscle growth. Think long distant runner.

Ectomorph

Mesomorph
Features: Broad chest and shoulders compared to hips, heavy bones, generally triangular. Think competitive swimmers.

Mesomorph

This is **not an excuse** to sit on the sofa and do nothing because you were made that way! It doesn't matter what shape you are, you still need to be healthy. If I use myself as an example, I am a "sort of" mesomorph. I am very broad in the shoulders with narrower hips, but just not tall enough for a classic mesomorph shape. I tend to put weight on around my top half. I used to long for elegant ladylike shoulders, but Praise Yahweh, I saw sense!!! I realised that I had been made that way for a reason. Skinny shoulders would not be much use for surfing and swimming, or shifting hay bales around the place, mucking out, and riding, I needed that upper body strength and power, so I thank Him for knowing best. I am 5'4" and weigh anything from 9st 10lbs to 10st 4lbs (136 – 144 lbs). My body fat is around 30% which isn't brilliant but is acceptable for a female of my age. This is the weight range I allow myself. We will look at range more closely when we look at maintenance. Suffice it to say here that this is the weight range I feel most comfortable with. If I start to creep up to my upper limit, I start focusing on what I am eating and my physical activity levels a little more conscientiously. I allow myself to be heavier in the winter as naturally you tend to eat more. It would be quite pointless for me to try to reach a weight that might be advised for my height because I have muscles and my body type dictates a heavier amount.

So, when you set your long term weight loss goals, be realistic. It may be that you have been a specific weight in the past that you were comfortable with. This is usually a good guide to initiate goal setting.

How Much Should I Be Eating?

Whichever way you want to go to lose or to gain, it is all about balance. The KEY is getting the balance right:

<u>**Energy Intake**</u>   Versus   <u>**Energy Output**</u>

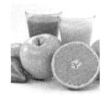   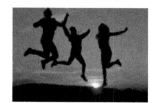

                                    Physical Activity /   Exercise
Food and Drink   Metabolism / Daily Activities
                                    Movement / Posture

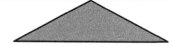

To keep your weight the same, Energy In has to equal Energy Out.

To lose weight, the Energy In has to be less than the Energy Out.

To gain weight, the Energy Out has to be less than the Energy In.

Based on the healthy eating guidelines we have already covered, you can now use the **Eatwell** plate by allocating numbers of portions to each food group. In this way, you maintain a healthy balance whilst also managing your weight.

Suggested portions based UK guidelines:

	For weight loss: Based on 1500-1800 calories	For weight gain:
Fruit and vegetables	7-8 portions	8+
Bread, rice, potatoes, pasta and other starchy foods	7-8 portions	8+
Milk and dairy	2 portions	3+ (avoiding high fats)
Meat, fish, eggs, beans and other non-dairy sources of protein	2 portions	3+ (avoiding high fats)
Spreading fats and oils, including all dressings and sauces	3 portions	3+ (good oils –poly/ monounsaturated)
High fat/high sugar including alcohol	100-200 kcal	200+ but with caution

Please note: For weight gain, food in general is not restricted, but care must be taken in consuming the right nutrients. Just because people are slim doesn't indicate that they are healthy.

Quick Ways of Measuring a Portion

Food Group	1 Portion =
Fruit and Vegetables	A double hand full
Carbohydrates - Bread, rice, potatoes, pasta, and other starchy foods	Approximately the size of your hand
Milk and Dairy - Cheese, milk, and yoghourt, and other dairy products	A small matchbox size 1 medium sized glass 1 small pot
Protein - Meat, fish, eggs, beans, and other non-dairy sources of protein	Approximately the size of your palm
Fats - Spreading fats and oils, including all dressings and sauces	1 teaspoon
Fat and Sugar - High fat/high sugar including alcohol	1 small glass wine 1 small chocolate bar
Fluids - Recommended: 8 large glasses of water per day. Tea and coffee may be included here.	

Weight Gain

Gaining weight for most people is not a problem. We are hard wired to survive and our bodies like to keep stores of surplus energy. For some people, however, this seems like an impossible task. Part of who we are in terms of shape and size is influenced by our genetic make up and body type. You will know people who appear to be able to eat anything and remain slim. I worked with a lovely gentleman as a personal training client who was 6'4" and 9 ½ stone (133 lbs). He was trying to get into the military and needed to put on just half a stone (7 lbs). He was incredibly fit and had already passed their initial fitness tests with flying colours. I saw how much he ate in a day, which was enough to satisfy a Sumo wrestler, and so it was a real challenge to add some poundage. He would actually sweat as he ate and you could almost see his body burning the calories. We spent a lot of time in the gym with the weights and added concentrated food drinks and plenty of peanut butter sandwiches into his meal planning. Up to the trials deadline we simply stopped all his running and martial arts, anything physical that might add to his calorie burn, and any activity that we didn't need for adding bulk. Finally, he put on sufficient weight, which was a huge relief all round, but it had been a real challenge. This is generally how hard it is to increase weight. Between metabolism, body type, and genetics, increasing weight can be a significant battle. Consider your family genetics. Are you all slim? If so, are you simply naturally slim, or are you actually underweight?

So, what can you do? Initially, I would suggest that you do exactly as I will suggest to those who are wanting to lose weight. Keep a truth and food diary for a week or so. There are some sample diary sheets later in the chapter. Compare your diary with the portion chart and check to see if what you are eating is sufficient. If not, then try to gradually either increase the number of portions you have at one meal, or, if you find eating this much at one time difficult, have the extra portions as snacks. If this isn't the case and you are eating plenty, and you are the only slim person in your family, then it might be worth having a check with your GP to see if everything is alright. If everything is in order and you get a clean bill of health, then it is all about trying to rebalance the scales, energy in versus energy out. Weight training and weight bearing exercises are good for building muscle. We will discuss this more fully in the next chapter, but suffice it to say here, that it does not mean that you will look like an elite bodybuilder, unless you want to and your genetics and body type allow you. Using weights and weight bearing exercises can be used simply to tone up and look more shapely or it can be used to actually build muscle. It is all down to the programme you are using. It can be a useful way of getting a few pounds on and having a bit more shape. Really have a close look at the foods you are eating and ensure that you are eating a good balance of foods. It might be that you eat till you are full, but most of it is on low fat, low calorie foodstuff. It is the quality and calorie value of the foods you eat that are important. For weight loss we look at pinching calories, in the way you cook, the foodstuffs you choose, the ingredients you use, etc. For weight gain it is exactly the same, but in reverse. It is important that you look at your shape and weight in a positive way

Long Term Weight Loss

One of the hardest parts of this long term weight loss programme is realising that it is more than just cutting the calories. Most people have been on a restrictive diet at some stage and so to be losing weight when the restrictions are no longer there, except that you are eating more healthily, is actually much harder. Due to there being less hard and fast rules, many people struggle with the fact that the choices remain under their control, rather than simply following a prescribed diet.

I am going to be quite firm here and suggest that unless you are seriously ready for change in this area, then you are wasting your time. When I run weight management courses, the first session is all about the readiness of each individual to change. I give them acres of forms to complete regarding their willingness and preparedness to change. Losing weight safely and effectively for the long term is a slow process and requires commitment and a willingness to change habits of a lifetime. It requires that you begin to think differently about food and that doesn't happen overnight.

Real weight loss also affects your identity, and for many, this is often a huge barrier to successful weight maintenance. If your identity is that of a large jolly person and everyone knows you as such, then to start losing weight requires an acceptance, by yourself, your family, and your friends, of the new shape and size. Believe it or not, I have actually had clients drop out of my weight management courses because their husbands or wives didn't like them being successful, looking better, and feeling more confident about themselves. So, pray about it and consider seriously, before you start, whether you are ready for the changes. It is about being disciplined in your decision making without putting yourself under enormous pressures to succeed, especially if you are also running a family, work, and whatever else. I am hoping that eating more healthily will involve the whole family anyway, so it can be brought to the family as a bit of a "project," if that helps. Keep in mind that it is His Temple.

Dieting vs Weight Loss Through Healthy Eating

For the majority of the people I see professionally, when asked, healthy eating equates to dieting. It is really important to understand that this programme is not about dieting. In fact, it is quite the opposite. It is about freeing you up from the dieting trap and about embracing eating healthy, portion control, and safe and effective long term weight loss. So, what are the differences?

The principal difference, and the one that makes the biggest distinction, is that dieting is generally based around quite regulated restrictions. Over the past years there have been an amazing assortment of diets from the quite bizarre to some that are quite dangerous to our health: ultra low calorie diets, ones that only allow you to eat protein and fat, high carbohydrate diets, low carbohydrate diets, blood group diets, food group diets, the celebrity diet, the beach diet, and all the ones in between. We are drawn to them because we are attracted to achieving quick results. In general, these restrictions are too much for any ordinary mortal to maintain and are simply not sustainable in the long term. This results in periods of high expectations at the start of the regime, *"This time it is going to work."* Then, as time progresses, your body demands that you feed it correctly. Motivation and self-discipline for the regime fade somewhat, and you start eating everything that comes in sight. "Planet Diet" is a very strange place to be. One day you are eating all sorts of different foodstuffs and generous quantities, and then on Monday (because all diets start on Mondays!) you start limiting your intake quite strictly. You are under enormous pressure to succeed. Whilst you stick to the diet regime, the weight falls off, and you receive praise from those around you, which in turn boosts your ego and spurs you on to keep the restrictions going.

This may, for some people, last for many months, but then you are invited out for a meal, or the family wants fast foods, or you have had a really miserable day at work, and you "break" your diet. This leads to guilt, which drives you to eat more because now you have, in your own mind, failed. More importantly, whilst you are restricting your food intake, your body has to respond. We are effectively hard wired to survive, and to survive when food is in short supply. So, when we restrict food intake, our metabolism does slow down. The jury is still out as to the degree to which this happens, but at present it is understood that it does slow down.

Also, if we are really restricting intake, and at the same time relying on diet alone to lose weight, with no physical exercise, then we will lose weight sure enough, but we will lose lean tissue as well as fat mass. The more lean tissue we have, the more calories we will burn because this is active tissue. Think muscle. If we lose this tissue, then when we start eating "normally" again we will simply put weight back on as stored fat, because, unless we start exercising, we won't regain the muscle tissue. This in turn creates a state of despondency, you loathe yourself and your failings and you spend the next few weeks beating yourself up. It is important to recognise that men also go through this cycle, but they tend not to be quite so outspoken about it.

The Diet Trap:

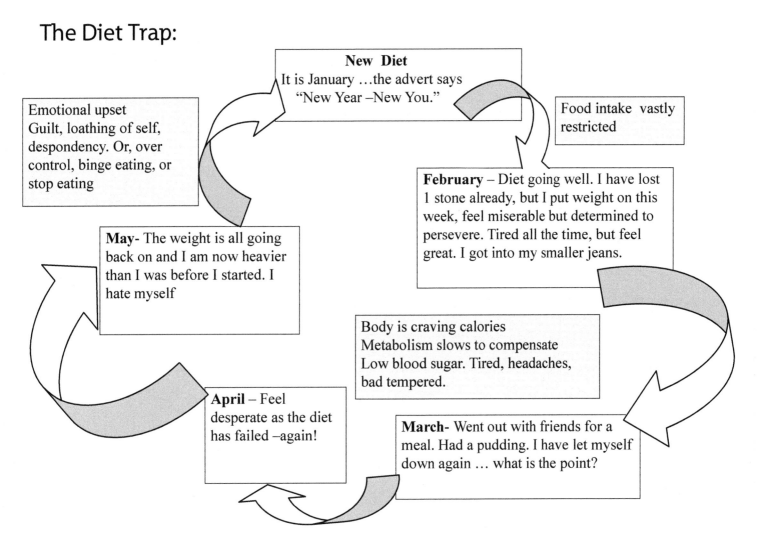

New Diet
It is January …the advert says
"New Year –New You."

Emotional upset
Guilt, loathing of self,
despondency. Or, over
control, binge eating, or
stop eating

Food intake vastly
restricted

February – Diet going well. I have lost
1 stone already, but I put weight on this
week, feel miserable but determined to
persevere. Tired all the time, but feel
great. I got into my smaller jeans.

May- The weight is all going
back on and I am now heavier
than I was before I started. I
hate myself

Body is craving calories
Metabolism slows to compensate
Low blood sugar. Tired, headaches,
bad tempered.

April – Feel
desperate as the diet
has failed –again!

March- Went out with friends for a
meal. Had a pudding. I have let myself
down again … what is the point?

Long Term Weight Loss: How?

Physiologically, your body can only lose around 2 lbs. of fat in around seven days. Anymore than that is going to be lean tissue and water. It is fat you want to lose and this can only be done slowly. I suggest that my clients aim for no more than 1 ½ lbs. per week. Slow, in this case, is excellent. If you have a substantial amount of weight to lose, then it may seem like a lifetime to lose the weight this slowly, BUT, I said that this was a different approach and this is the way that will keep the weight off. We are talking about for the rest of your life, so be strong and persevere. I want to instill hope in you that you can achieve this, and you can. It is, of course, also about changing your eating habits, lifestyle, and possibly your identity, and these also need time.

The reality of this is as follows:

o 1lb. of fat is equivalent to 3,500 Kcals.

o To lose 1 pound of fat per week, you need to set the balance that you are 3,500 Kcals below your energy expenditure.

o (To gain weight, you need to be way above this figure.)

o This sounds like a lot, but if you split it down:

> If you divide 3,500 Kcals ÷ 7days = 500 Kcals /day
>
> =250 Kcals less in food and 250 Kcals increase in calorie burning physical activity.

Check your portions and sizes of portions using your diaries, which we will be looking at shortly. The portions I have quoted are for a range from 1500-1800 Kcals. If you know you are really active and have a physically demanding job, then these figures need to be adjusted accordingly. Recent research is suggesting that a faster weight loss can be effective, but as this book goes to press, this work has not been substantiated.

Ten Keys to Success

1. Securing your support network

2. Being ready to change

3. Setting SMARTT goals

4. Keeping records/diaries

5. Staying motivated

6. Controlling portions

7. Reducing fat and sugar intake

8. Understanding weight maintenance

9. Addressing emotional eating

10. Increasing physical activity

1. Securing Your Support Network

Having the support of friends and family is extremely important. They will keep you going when you are flagging, will allow you to lean on them when you need it, and will give you a kick in the right direction when you start to feel sorry for yourself. It doesn't necessarily need to be close friends or indeed any of your family.

Some people prefer to be with others that have a better understanding of what they are going through. So if you can get a small group together who all want to join you, then you have each other. Why not organise a group that goes to the gym or goes walking on a regular basis? This can be added to a healthy weight loss programme. It gets you out in the fresh air and is terrific fellowship.

2. Being Ready to Change

If you need to, re-read Chapter 2 to familiarise yourself again with the cycle of change. I am hoping that, in some way, as you have been reading through the chapters, it has instilled a new enthusiasm and hope for a healthier lifestyle.

3. Setting S.M.A.R.T.T. Goals

If you are ready, then the first task is to set your SMARTT goals. Return to Chapter 3, read it through if necessary, and use the examples provided to help you establish clear and realistic goals. You need to identify a *long term goal*. Where do you want to be in six months time? Now break this down into bite size and achievable targets for your *medium goals* and your *short term goals*. Record these and keep them somewhere handy, so that you can refer to them when you need a gentle reminder of where you are heading.

4. Keeping Records / Diaries

Daily Truth Diary

The daily truth diary is an essential part of the process of planning and change.

5-10 minutes every day will help you to identify the areas that require special attention. The diary will also be a vital reference point for you to examine and make comparisons in terms of change and improvements for you individually. Ideally, you will have your diary with you at all times. This is frequently a challenge to begin with, but after the first few days most people report that they "couldn't manage without it." Your diary is a record of *everything* that you have eaten and drank. This includes **all snacks, drinks, broken biscuits (cookies), and left overs**.

Many people find this extremely difficult to start with as they often feel guilty and embarrassed. The important thing is that you discover what your difficult areas are, and the diary helps to identify these more specifically. Also, we often forget exactly what and how much we eat in a day and the diary does help us to actually see it as it is. We call this the "Eye to Mouth Gap." It is important also to record why you needed to eat. Was it from stomach hunger, meal time, boredom, anxiety, feeling upset, or for a social reason? The more information you can record, the easier it will be to identify potential barriers to weight loss.

Activity Diary

"If you fail to plan, you plan to fail!"

Plan your activities at the beginning of the week. Try and do something active for an hour a day each day. This doesn't necessarily have to be planned exercise, but could include things like walking to the shops instead of taking the car. Don't allow yourself to negotiate with this set plan, you will already be expert at talking yourself out of doing things…..don't listen!!

Record how it went, and how you felt before, during, and after. What was your time, and at what effort level were you working, on a scale from 1-10?

Food Diary

This is a good starting point to identify whether or not you are eating the correct portions and getting the right balance. In this diary, you simply record what you are eating and drinking and allocate these into the correct food categories. Refer back to the portions and portion sizes at the beginning of this chapter and check to see what and how much you are eating.

On the next few pages are some examples of what your diaries may look like. Cut out and keep these (or make copies) if they are helpful to get you started.

Food Truth Diary

Time	Food/Drink	Snacks	Amount	Situation Where? Why? What mood were you in?

Activity Diary

Week:

	Activity?	Time?	Where?	Who was there?
Monday				
Tuesday				
Wednesday				
Thursday				
Friday				
Saturday				
Sunday				

Week:

	Activity?	Time?	Where?	Who was there?
Monday				
Tuesday				
Wednesday				
Thursday				
Friday				
Saturday				
Sunday				

Food Diary

Date:

Time	Food	Category	Amount/ Portion

Summary of daily food intake:	Number of Portions	Portions under / Over allowance?
1. Bread, cereal, rice, pasta, potatoes		
2. Fruits and vegetables		
3. Meat, fish, and protein alternatives		
4. Dairy, milk, yoghourt, cheese		
5. Fats and oils		
6. High fat /sugar foods, including alcohol		

5. Staying Motivated

Anyone can lose weight? If you were offered $10,000 to lose 10% body weight, could you do it?

Motivation—if only you could bottle it!

Motivation - It begins, maintains, and influences our behaviour. It is drive, passion, tenacity, and desire to achieve certain goals. It is zest, enthusiasm, and inner power—your get up and go.

There are numerous theories regarding motivation, but for our purposes, two are relevant:

❖ **Extrinsic motivation:** This is motivation from outside the individual, such as winning a cup, making money, social recognition, or praise from our superiors or peers.

❖ **Intrinsic motivation:** Self-motivation that emanates from within us, the individual. Research suggests that this intrinsic motivation is likely to last longer than that generated from extrinsic sources. So, the importance of you as an individual getting to the point at which you yourself want to change will also influence your own drive and motivation.

Many issues may impact our levels of motivation. These include: stress, illness, believing that we are incapable of a certain task, procrastination, and tiredness. You will be only too aware that simply having a desire to do something doesn't necessarily provide you with sufficient drive to actually start to achieve it. Lack of both enthusiasm and the motivation to take initial action, or to maintain it, can be quite debilitating and may lead to feelings of frustration, dissatisfaction, and sometimes deep unhappiness. The "should" word appears frequently when we lack that little bit of extra push. "I really should go for a walk, but it's pouring down." Weight loss and fitness regimes are a pertinent and perfect example of instances where initial enthusiasm and energy soon wane.

All is not doom and despair!

These things will help:

❖ Set SMARTT goals and have a clear vision of where and what you want to achieve. This is key to motivation.

❖ Be honest about how much you desire the changes.

❖ Don't allow negative thinking or procrastination – Just get out there!!!

❖ Read books and magazine articles that inspire. Running and fitness magazines, along with those that have new healthy eating recipes in them, always have inspiring articles in them. You don't have to be an athlete or a chef to read them. Just be inspired.

❖ Visualise what it will be like and how you will feel when you reach your goal. Keep this picture constantly in your mind.

❖ Focus and dwell on your goal. Have it in your mind's eye when, for example, you go shopping!

❖ Write positive notes and Bible verses to yourself and put them where you can see them on the fridge door and your mirror.

❖ And finally, remember why you are doing this. If you need to, re-read the Bible studies and reflect on where you are right now.

"Instead of giving myself reasons why I can't, I give myself reasons why I can."

(Author unknown)

6. Controlling Portions

✓ Check your portions and portion sizes and stick to them.

✓ If you are feeling peckish because you are genuinely stomach hungry, then have some fruit.

We live today in an environment of excess where extra large portions are the norm. Unfortunately, we have become used to this state of affairs and basically we all eat too much. If you have the time and you want to have a go at this, get the portion chart out and put out exactly the amount of food that you need to be eating in a day. Many years ago, I attended one of my first nutrition courses. We all had to run a presentation at the end of the course, and the only one that I really remember is this lady demonstrating how much 1500 Kcalories looked like as a plate of food.....It didn't look like very much! This image is still with me today and it works a treat. We do not need the amount of food that we are all consuming. Having said all that, it is a difficult task to suddenly cut your portion sizes dramatically, and it *is* a question of pinching calories. Just be aware and alert that you are looking to reduce the energy going in. If you gradually reduce the servings, it will have bring the desired results. Eat slowly and allow yourself to feel full.

7. Reducing Fat and Sugar Intake

We looked previously at hidden fats and sugars. Similarly to the portion sizes, many of the products we eat today are high in fat, sugar, and salt. I have spent hours trawling the shelves of supermarkets trying to find foodstuffs that do not contain at least one of these, and found only a few. So this is not an easy task when you are trying to cut down. If you focus on your portion sizes and make up the bulk of your meals from complex carbohydrates and fruit and vegetables, then this can make satisfying savings on your fat and sugar content.

If you can, and you have the time, it is really helpful if you spend a bit of time reading the food labels of products you commonly buy. Use the **"A Lot"** and **"A Little"** lists on page 98 and just quickly check to see if any of your foods are on the "A Lot" list. Clever marketing and packaging can easily betray the reality of what actually lurks within foodstuffs. It doesn't necessarily follow that labels suggesting that the items are healthy actually are. As an example, have a look at some of the smoothies and flapjacks that are frequently packaged and marketed as," organic," "natural," or coming from "mother nature" and just check how much sugar they contain. Without getting too clinical about this, you will soon learn which products are healthier.

If you are cooking meals, then consider adapting some of your recipes to cut down on the overall fats and sugars. This is easily done and is quite often tastier and cheaper.

Following are a couple of recipes as examples:

Lasagne (serves 4)

Original recipe	Modifications
2 tbsp vegetable oil	Nil for dry fry or a teaspoon of olive oil/grapeseed
2 onions	
1 carrot chopped	Add broccoli and favourite vegetables
1clove garlic	
450g minced beef	250g of lean mince plus spinach, red kidney beans
400g tomatoes tinned	Fresh or tinned but with no added sugars
2tbsp tomato puree	
300ml beef stock	
12 sheets lasagne	
50g parmesan	Use whole meal bread crumbs for topping instead

Cheese sauce:

75g butter	Low-fat cooking margarine
75g plain flour	
1 1/2 pts of milk	Semi-skimmed
50g Cheddar cheese	Half fat cheese

Preparation:

Grease a three litre oven-proof dish.

Heat oil in a large pan and fry onions, garlic, and carrot.

Add minced beef and fry for 3-4 minutes until brown.

Stir in tomatoes, tomato puree, stock, and seasoning.

Simmer and cover for 30 minutes.

Melt butter, add flour and stir for 1 min.
Remove from heat and add milk.
Bring to boil until it thickens.
Season and add cheese.

Preheat oven 350 F
Layer - 4 sheets lasagne.
    Cover with half meat sauce,
        then third cheese sauce.
Repeat layers, finishing with lasagne,
    cheese sauce, and parmesan.
Bake for 45 minutes.

Modifications

Use a non-stick pan.

Dry fry or use a small amount of olive oil.

Drain fat after browning as above.

Lightly steam spinach and lightly boil extra vegetables, broccoli, etc. Keep to side.

Halve amounts for cheese sauce.

Layer meat with vegetables and then cheese sauce.

Sprinkle with bread crumbs.

Chili Con Carne (serves 4-5)

Original recipe	Modifications
2 tbsp cooking oil	Reduce amount of oil. Dry fry. Use mono/polyunsaturated oil
1 onion	
1 clove garlic-crushed	
1 lb minced beef	Use lean minced beef.
1 tbsp flour	
8 oz can tomatoes	Use fresh tomatoes.
8 oz can kidney beans	
2 tbsp tomato puree	Miss out or use fresh tomatoes.
pinch marjoram	(1 tbsp puree = 3 gms sugar)
chili powder	
seasoning	

Preparation:

Place oil, garlic, and beef in saucepan until minced beef is browned.

Stir in flour.

Add can tomatoes, tomato puree, chili powder, and marjoram.

Add beans and cook for 5 minutes.

Serve with rice.

Dry cook or use very light oil. Drain.

Omit tomato puree.

Serve with brown rice and green salad.

8. Understanding Weight Maintenance

Weight maintenance is described as a less than 3% change in bodyweight after weight loss. Weight maintenance is just as much a challenge as weight loss and should be seen as part of the overall programme. It is also a significant achievement!

If you are losing weight steadily, at some point you may well reach a plateau. Plateaus are not a sign of failure, but an indicator that your body is adjusting to the extra physical activity and healthy eating.

Step 1. Identify what weight range you are comfortable with. It might not be one that you previously found acceptable.

Step 2. Recognise that your body adjusts really quickly to your new healthy lifestyle and it is not that you have "failed." It may be that it is time to revisit the goals that you set initially and to adjust them accordingly. We often set goals too low in the first place and we need to keep up with our achievements.

Step 3. Accept that maintaining your weight doesn't have the same buzz as losing it. To have the tape measure slowly record how much slimmer your waist is, or to have work colleagues comment on how well you are looking helps you to remain focused and motivated.

Step 4. Adjust to the fact that maintaining your weight is not time limited.

Step 5 Keep challenging your body in different ways by changing the amount, level, and type of exercise that you do. Also, keep an eye on what you are eating. If you are losing weight regularly it is easy to become complacent. Then it can be really hard going initially when you reach the plateaus. Once you learn to manage these, however, and to reset your goals and you restart losing the weight, they will become less and less of a hurdle

Weight maintenance is key to successful long term weight management. You will soon find that you can still lose weight even though you are not on a restrictive "diet." You will come across weight plateaus as your body adjusts to the increases in physical activity and as it adapts to your new healthy eating regime. See weight maintenance as part of keeping your weight at a healthy level. Monitor your weight at regular intervals and if necessary, just consider focusing on what you are eating and your level of exercise. For example:

- Fitting in a little more physical activity, 20 minutes in the lunch break.
- Keeping a food diary again for a couple of weeks to help refocus on food choices.
- Varying the exercise routine as the body may well have become more adapted and efficient, and therefore, will use less calories than before for a given workload.

STAY FOCUSED!!!

9. Addressing Emotional Eating

Re-read the section on emotional eating. It might be that in getting this far, you have realised that your emotions are more influenced by food than you thought. Do not let your feelings and emotions trip you up. Bring them to Adonai in prayer, and try and get to the root of what is causing the chaos and focus on the renewing of your mind. Again, if you need help and support, ask.

10. Increasing Physical Activity

Whilst weight loss can be achieved slowly by eating healthily and portion control, we need to consider a healthy lifestyle as a whole and that involves physical activity of some sort. Increasing your physical activity of course also helps to burn calories and contributes to weight loss. We were made to run and jump and sit and stand and leap and crawl and walk. So we are much better off when we are moving around. Being active helps to maintain in good order our respiratory, circulatory, and musculoskeletal systems, as well as our ninds and emotions. It is good for us. We will look at physical activity in detail in the next chapter.

The Difficult Scriptures About Weight Loss

I am including a few words here regarding the many Scriptures that deal with such subjects as self-control, greed, gluttony, etc. It comes up time and again, usually when the subject being discussed is weight loss, which is why I am suggesting its relevance here.

Whilst it is important that we are aware what Scripture is telling us, it might not be an appropriate time to study these. If you are still full of self-loathing, feeling guilty, or are someone who condemns yourself, then I suggest you leave these until you have sorted those other issues out. If, however, you are really comfortable with yourself and really know that you need a more disciplined approach, then the following verses might help you to paint a clearer picture.

Remember that:

"There is now no condemnation for those who are in Christ Jesus" (Romans 8:1 NIV).

Do not forget God's promises to us when reading these verses. We have to understand before we can act. Ask the Holy Spirit to teach you. Begin to see and understand what, how, and why God wants you to act. ALL things are possible to those that love Christ.

Look up the definition of the following words:

Greed:

Greedy:

Gluttony:

Idolatry:

Greed:

Please read:

Proverbs 1:19

Psalm 10:3

Ephesians 4:17-21

Gluttony is a form of idolatry:

Isaiah 22: 12-14

Ephesians 5:1-20

1 Corinthians 10:6-10

James 5:5

Gluttony is closely linked with drunkeness:

Exodus 32:6

Judges 9:27

Proverbs 20:1

Isaiah 5:11

Romans 14:21

Gluttony the destructive forces of:

Proverbs 15:27

　　　23:20-21

　　　28:7

　　　28:25

Ecclesiastes 6:7

Warnings against gluttony:

Proverbs 23:1-2

Luke12:15, 12:19-20 and 21:34

Ephesians 5:3

Colossians 3:5-16

Galatians 5:19-21

1 Corinthians 5;4-11

1 Peter 4:3-4

Gluttony may be paralleled with neglect. We may not be a glutton,

but we may fail on the upkeep of our "building."

Please read:

2 Peter 2:19

"The Lord is gracious and compassionate, slow to anger and rich in love. The Lord is good to all; he has

compassion on all he has made."

Psalm 145:8-9

Chapter Eight – Physical Activity

Introduction

We currently exist in what is now referred to as an obesogenic environment, in other words, one that has an impact on our weight, and supports us in being overweight. Think of your own environment: you can park directly outside the supermarket; you can get escalators to the second floor of every building; you drive your children to the door everywhere for safety; most of you have jobs that you sit down to all day; you are surrounded by high energy, low nutrient food; and the majority of you take very little or no exercise. If we go out for a meal we expect the pasta dish to come in what our grandparents would have considered a serving dish, and, if we don't get a bowl of chips on the side, we think we are hard done by. We effectively live in a world of excess, where food is abundant, and we do not have to really think too hard about obtaining it. Whilst I am exaggerating the point here, I am trying to highlight the need for a possible rethink of our lifestyles. We are so accustomed to this lifestyle that, unfortunately, we often fail to recognise what it is doing to our health.

Consider everything we have looked at so far and ask yourself these questions: Why do we need a healthy lifestyle, what does it involve, how do we go about changing to healthier options, what barriers do we have to address? In this chapter, we are going to consider **physical activity**, which is key to achieving a healthy lifestyle. As I hope to make clear, this doesn't necessarily mean pounding for hours on the treadmill at the local gym or pumping iron until you can't move. It is more about being more active because you want to be, doing activities that are meaningful and beneficial to your health, and simply getting out and enjoying His Creation. Following is a very simplistic guide to increasing your physical activity because to add detail would entail several volumes. There is a plethora of books and information on specific training regimes and exercise programmes for you to study once you are ready. Here, we will simply look at some of the ways in which you can get started and will underline some of the basic principles of physical activity and exercise.

IMPORTANT

It is vitally important that if you are in *any* doubt as to whether or not you should increase your physical activity, you should first consult your family doctor. This will also give you the confidence to set your goals appropriately, be they walking up the stairs or climbing the highest mountain. Even if you are young and apparently healthy, it is a good idea to check with your doctor if you can. I would NEVER take anyone on as a client without first getting them to complete a medical questionnaire.

Physical Activity: Why?

Long Term Benefits:

   ✓ The heart muscles become stronger and the heart becomes more efficient.

   ✓ Heart recovery improves after exertion.

   ✓ Resting heart rate is lowered.

   ✓ Blood pressure is reduced.

   ✓ Your breathing mechanism becomes more efficient.

   ✓ Overall fitness is increased.

   ✓ Number of capillaries and blood flow is increased.

   ✓ Number of red blood cells (increased oxygen carrying capacity) is increased.

   ✓ Size and number of myofibrils may increase, helping your muscles to become stronger and improving movement.

   ✓ Muscle fibre recruitment is increased, which means muscles become stronger and more efficient.

   ✓ Bone mass is enhanced.

   ✓ Ability to process oxygen in the cells and to release energy is increased.

   ✓ Ability to store glycogen is increased.

   ✓ Ability to utilise fat is increased.

               These mean that you are controlling your blood sugar better and utilising stored energy better.

Plus You Will Have: (depending on your physical activity level and type)

         o   Increased lean body mass

         o   Reduced body fat

         o   Decreased cholesterol levels

         o   Increased good cholesterol

         o   Decreased fat levels in blood

         o   Reduced stress and anxiety

         o   Improved insulin response and blood sugar control

What is Physical Activity?

We often see physical activity as being interchangeable with exercise. For our purposes I would like to be a little more specific. **Physical activity**, as it is truly defined, involves bodily movement produced by the muscles that results in energy expenditure. In other words it is more of an umbrella term that involves activity. This could be anything from vacuuming the floor, to running for a bus, peeling the potatoes, or walking to work. Sitting and standing even involve some energy expenditure, and for some people this is quite a task. If you experience conditions like arthritis and you are in constant pain, then simply standing for any time is often a greater effort than most people would expend walking.

Exercise

On the other hand, exercise sits under the umbrella of physical activity and involves elements such as planning, structure, and motivation. It is focused on both the improvement and maintenance of selected aspects of physical fitness and generally involves repetitive movement, for example, a prescribed exercise programme at the gym. The body will respond to the demands that you put on it and in prescribing programmes, the instructor or coach uses their knowledge and skill in designing specific regimes that will get the outcomes you desire.

Our overall **fitness** is about how able our body is at coping with the demands put on it. This may include our physical, nutritional, medical, mental, and emotional fitness.

Functional Fitness is the basic fitness we need in order to achieve our everyday tasks, doing what we call ADL's in occupational therapy parlance, "activities of daily living."

Physical Fitness is a part of **fitness** and describes the capability of your body's circulation, respiratory, and musculoskeletal systems to function optimally with the demands you put on it. For example: Do you get breathless going upstairs, or can you go up with no effort two at a time?

Physical fitness is made up of the following components:

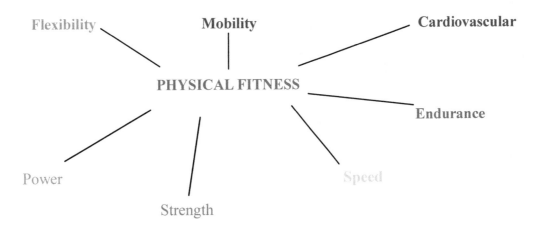

Cardiovascular fitness: How well do your heart and lungs work? Can you climb the stairs easily, or do you huff and puff? Can you run for the bus without getting out of breath?

Strength and Endurance: How easily do you lift a weighted load? How far can you carry that load? Can you carry all your shopping all the way to the car?

Speed: How fast can you run for the bus?

Power: A mix of strength and speed. How easily does the sprinter leave his blocks? How easily does the weight lifter start the lift? How easily do you find the stop/start in your local football/soccer game?

Mobility and Flexibility: Mobility is how far you can move that joint through a range of movement easily and with no effort. This is your "normal" range of movement. Flexibility is how far you can move that joint through a greater range of movement. In its extreme, think of a ballet dancer or a gymnast who, through training, can move their limbs through a remarkable range of movement. The more flexible you are, the less likely you are to suffer injuries. For example: If my hamstrings and calves are as flexible as they can be, then when I use my hip joints and knees kicking a football, I am less likely to tear my hamstring as it is used to traveling through this range.

Pre-Activity Checklist

Before you start any physical activity programme, it is vitally important that you are not "at risk." As a fitness instructor, I would want to know a lot about you in terms of medical history and presenting conditions prior to taking you on as a client. For example: Do you have diabetes, any injuries, back problems? Do you get dizzy when you stand up, is your breathing alright, do you have high blood pressure, do you have low blood pressure, has your family got a history of heart problems, do you smoke, do you drink and how much, how often?

All of these need to be checked off prior to increasing your physical activity, especially if you plan to incorporate a planned exercise session or two into your new regime. Anyone who is responsible for instructing exercise has various risk stratifications that they will utilise to screen clients. In the same way, it is important that if you are in any doubt that increasing your physical activity level may be detrimental to your health, you need to first pass it by your doctor. You will also need to consider any specific precautions that you need to take regarding your condition.

In Britain, if you need support to get you started, your doctor can refer you to an Exercise on Prescription course, which are usually run by your local council sports facility. Once you have attended these courses, you will be much better informed and have more confidence to carry on independently. You will also learn how to monitor yourself correctly so that your physical activities may be both safe and effective.

What If I Find Physical Activity Too Difficult?

There are many people for whom just getting from the chair to standing is an effort. If, for example you have a respiratory condition, arthritis, multiple sclerosis, osteoporosis, or obesity, then it is about focusing on what activities may both help and improve your ability to manage your condition and your quality of life. Depression and low mood frequently accompany many of these conditions, and being more active can often have a much greater impact than just improving your physical fitness.

It is vitally important that you ask your consultant if you could consider increasing your physical activity level. If the answer is yes, then it is not only about choosing appropriate activities but also about seeking out the right support network. A useful start is to look at local support groups that may well have exercise classes running that are suitable. I have a couple of friends who attend the local MS support group swimming sessions. Water-based activities are a useful option where non-weight-bearing activities are indicated.

You may also find that you are better at certain times of the day, and so try to incorporate your new activity into these times. It may also be helpful to access the organisations that specialise in your condition, as they will tell you what activities are best and also what level you need to be working.

Pacing is key! Just because you are feeling good today, doesn't mean you do everything like a bull in a china shop because, as you know, this will only result in you being laid low for days. The key is to start really slowly, gradually increasing your activity levels. If you have no negative response to this level, then continue to increase the effort very slowly. If you are laid low with a flare up or fatigue, then rest, as your body knows best, but then you will have heard this a thousand times already!

How Do I Increase My Physical Activity?

Increasing your physical activity will aid weight loss, as you will be burning calories instead of storing them. Physical fitness is about being the best we can physically and maintaining the systems that run our body. It is about caring for this "jar of clay" or "the Temple" and about keeping it all in working order. Different forms of exercise will focus on different aspects. For example: If you want to have better cardiovascular health, that is, your heart and lungs, then simply doing a stretch and relaxation class isn't going to achieve this as it is not making the heart and lungs work hard enough. Because of this varied response of the body to the demands we put on it, we need to know exactly what it is we want to achieve. There are two questions you need to ask yourself:

1. **What are my specific goals regarding my physical fitness?**

2. **What do I enjoy doing?**

Your goals could be anything from wanting to run a marathon to simply wanting to be able to complete the household chores without becoming exhausted. I am currently running a class aimed at the older client. We focus on strengthening and balance exercises to help avoid falls and to make getting around easier, as well as a short section that is aerobic in order to improve their endurance which, in turn, will improve components, such as their standing tolerance. I put on a bit of old time dance music and they all reminisce of their younger days, so not only are we working on physical fitness, but we all go away feeling much better after having had a really good natter and a bit of a social. When setting your goals, therefore, it is about all of these aspects. If you are not going to enjoy whatever it is you choose to focus on, then it will become something of a chore and you are not going to want to maintain your regime.

Key to Increasing Physical Activity is in Setting Your S.M.A.R.T.T. Goals

Do you want to:

- o   Lose weight?
- o   Just get fitter?
- o   Climb the stairs without getting breathless?
- o   Get fitter to play soccer/tennis?
- o   Improve your heart health?
- o   Train for a local charity run?

In setting your SMARTT goals it is useful to have a significant end goal in mind. We considered this in Chapter 3 when we looked at how to set SMARTT goals. If I am simply exercising for exercise sake, then it will soon lose its appeal, but in order to keep you focused and motivated, especially if you are new to physical activity, then aim to do something that you have always wanted to have a go at. Charity events are a great way of achieving this, be they the local sponsored walk or jumping out of an aeroplane. Focusing on others rather than yourself helps to keep you going when you are having your off days, as all you have to do is think of those for whom you are doing it, and it will also reinforce the benefits of a healthy lifestyle. Don't feel excluded if you are managing an illness. Set yourself your own achievable challenges and simply go for it. Many charity events accommodate wheelchair users and less able competitors. **So be there! Praise Him. Go Enjoy!**

Step 1

What do you want to achieve?

Step 2

Consider what you really enjoy doing.

Step 3

Set your SMARTT goals that are meaningful to you for:

Long term

Medium term

Short term

Refer back to Chapter 3 (page 63). Use the examples to really look at all the aspects of setting and achieving your goals. For example: How will you know when you have achieved your goals?

If you are working through this in a small group, then plan these together and encourage each other within the group. Why not get a 5-a-side team together, a church walking group, or badminton. It doesn't matter what you choose as long as it will challenge your body in a way that will result in improvement. Whatever it is, the key is to enjoy it ......

The majority of people will be looking to improve their general fitness and this involves all of the aspects of physical fitness. If we now look at each of the components that make up **physical fitness,** you can then decide to mix and match your activities in order to achieve your goals. We will also consider both **posture** and **core stability and strength** in this section as these elements are foundational to our physical fitness and will be covered when we consider **Muscular Strength and Endurance (MSE).** KEY for weight loss, as well as for all around fitness, is to combine both cardiovascular (CV) fitness (heart and lungs), and muscular strength and endurance (MSE) work. (Both of these will be explained in detail later.) This way you are challenging the body in a number of ways, and are burning off extra calories. Healthy eating alone without exercise is a long haul if you are wanting to shed the pounds. Ideally, you need to be considering a mixture of all of the following types of exercise preceded by an adequate warm up session.

Warming Up

Prior to starting any planned physical activity, you need to be warmed up. The warm up helps prepare the body for what is to come and also reduces the likelihood of injury. It also gets you in the right frame of mind and helps you focus on your activity. If your body is warm, your muscles and joints move more easily. Think of the sticky stuff you use to stick things on the wall. If it is cold it snaps easily, but when you warm it up it is more pliable and you can stretch it out. This is effectively what happens to our muscles when we warm them up. Likewise, we need to raise our heart rate slowly so that we don't get an abnormal change by suddenly putting it under too much load.

Depending on what you are going to do will determine the warm up. If I am taking a group out walking, I generally get them to walk actively for 10 minutes, whilst doing some extra little fun exercises like skipping, raising up on tip toes to warm the calves up, and lifting the knees up.

The jury is still out as to whether or not pre-exercise stretching is beneficial. It really depends on the group I have as to whether or not I include them. If I do, it is usually after about ten minutes of warm ups that we will briefly stretch our calves, quadriceps, and hamstrings, but we also try to keep moving between each stretch, by doing a few squats to challenge the legs and so that we don't cool down again. (Please see later notes on stretching exercises.)

If you are going to be doing resistant work, then it is just as important to be warmed up properly. A ten minute active walk around the block followed by squats to warm the legs up is a good start. Performing exercises utilising the big quadriceps muscles will help to raise the heart rate. Kick your heels to your bottom to warm up the hamstrings and then do a few calf raises by lifting up onto tippy toes. Knee lifts could also be included here. Make big circles with your arms to mobilise your shoulder joints, and bend the elbows touching your hands to your shoulders in a bicep curl. Incorporate stretches for the back, arms, hamstrings, hip flexors, calves, and quadriceps (please see below). I suggest around a ten minute warm up, but if you think you need longer take it. When you are just starting out, this can almost be your workout, but it doesn't matter. If I am doing a run, then I need around twenty minutes before I feel comfortable enough to really get going.

Cardiovascular Fitness

Cardiovascular (CV) fitness is all about your heart and lungs. Your heart is a muscle that needs to be worked in order to keep in its best of health just like all the other muscles. As we train, the circulatory system becomes better at extracting oxygen and providing energy for our muscles to work, as our capillaries improve their network. The heart itself becomes stronger and more efficient at pumping the blood around the body, and we begin to notice that our everyday tasks and exercise programme become easier, and that we are more comfortable when we exert ourselves. In actuality, increasing our physical activity in a way that makes the heart and lungs work harder can improve our cardiovascular fitness. The activity chosen has to effectively raise both your heart rate and your breathing whilst remaining within safe levels. Some examples would be: walking, washing the floor, gardening, running, swimming, cycling, dancing, going up and down stairs. Doing sufficient CV activity, at the correct level, will help to burn calories and balance your energy input and output. The more you do, the more energy you burn.

There are three different energy systems that work when we are active. Think of them as the start up system, the aerobic system, which means with oxygen, and finally, the anaerobic system—without oxygen. These different systems come into play when we work at different levels. "Aerobics," as a class format, came about because, in general, you work at a level that challenges the aerobic energy system. This means that your body is working at a level that can readily supply the oxygen it requires and keep the muscles fuelled with energy. As you increase the intensity of the activity, your body begins to switch to the anaerobic system, basically, because the aerobic system can no longer meet the demands you are putting on it. The body starts to use a system that can still supply energy to the working muscles but is not reliant on oxygen for its delivery, thus anaerobic, without oxygen. In this latter system, lactic acid is a by-product, and when it begins to build up, you begin to feel a dull ache in the muscles. This is a rather simplistic way of looking at it, as the body doesn't suddenly switch over to a different system. It is not possible to sustain this anaerobic intensity for very long, so high intensity training has to be carefully managed. If you ever want to work at this higher level, then read up about interval training, as it is a very achievable way to increase both intensity and effort.

How Do I Know When I Am Doing Enough?

The key to **cardiovascular** activities is that it needs to be at a level that will challenge you as an individual. Without having all the clinical equipment you would need to work these out accurately, there are a number of ways you can monitor how hard you are working.

One way of doing this is to record your heart rate and to calculate what are called your **target heart rate (THR) zones**. These are calculated as a percent of your **maximum heart rate (MHR)**. You may have seen the calculation that suggests you use the calculation 220 minus your age. This is far too generalised, and I suggest that if you want to work with a slightly more accurate reading, you could use what is known as the **Karvonen formula**. This is the one I use for my own clients in conjunction with the **rate of perceieved exertion (RPE) scale,** which we will look at shortly. The **Karvonen Formula** also incorporates your resting heart rate and can be used as a helpful guide for assessing your activity level.

For your **resting heart rate**, you need to be "at rest." When I take my own, I take it just after I have gotten out of bed, before I have been up and down stairs. I suggest that you sit quietly for 10 minutes and just relax. Place your index and middle fingers on the wrist of the opposite hand, that has its palm facing up. You can count the beats for 30 seconds and then multiply by two.

Karvonen Formula

Age maximum heart rate (AMHR):	220 – Your Age = A
AMHR minus resting heart rate (RHR):	A- RHR = B (Heart rate reserve HRR)
To calculate lower target training zone:Eg 65%	= B x 65 % = C
To calculate upper target training zone: Eg 75%	= B x 75% = D
Now add back in your RHR	
Lower target training zone = C + RHR	Upper target training zone = D + RHR

For the above to be applicable, ideally you will require a heart rate monitor. In order to ensure you are getting a training effect, you need to be working within these targeted heart rate zones.

BUT, if I am training someone, I take far more into consideration and use these simply as a guide. I meet many individuals who have accurately calculated their target heart rate zones, but are working way below, or above what they should be. You need to also take into account how your body responds to exercise, how fit you are, what level is safe for you to be working at, what you are wanting to achieve, endurance or speed, how well you are, how your heart is, whether you are seriously overweight. As a *very* rough guide, if you are out of condition and just starting out, then you need to be looking at a range of 60-70% AMHR, even lower initially. If you are reasonably active and there are no complications, then you can be aiming for 65 - 75% to get you started.

Rate of Perceived Exertion (RPE) Scale

A far simpler way, and one that is just as effective for our purposes, is the **rate of perceived exertion (RPE) scale.** There are a number of versions of this around that can all be credited to a gentleman called Gunner A.V. Borg in his article, "Psychophysical Bases of Perceived Exertion" in *Medicine and Science in Sports and Exercise,* 1982 (Vol. 14, No. 5, pp. 377– 381). You may have seen ones that cover a 20 point scale. The one I use is adapted from this and based on 10 points. It is very simple, but equally effective.

It is basically asking you what effort level you perceive you are working at:

Perceived Exertion:	RPE Scale	*Approx.* % of MHR
I am not exercising:	1	
I am exercising very little:	2	
I am exercising, but I am comfortable:	3	
I still feel comfortable, but I'm getting quite warm:	4	60%
I'm working hard now, but I can still hold a conversation:	5	65%
I can still talk to you, but it is getting much harder:	6	70 - 75%

Perceived Exertion:	RPE Scale	*Approx.* % of MHR
It is too hard to talk and exercise:	7	
I'm now well out of my comfort zone:	8	
I'm working extremely hard:	9	
I'm going to have to stop soon:	10	Reaching MHR

In order to be effective, you need to be exercising at a level that you perceive around RPE 5-6. If I am working with a client, I ask them how they feel and if they are still talking, but with short pauses, then this is around the 5-6 level. If, however, you are very unfit and become easily short of breath, drop this to RPE 3-4 until you feel that it is becoming easier.

How Long Should My Activity Last to Reach CV Fitness?

Guidelines for the length of time you need to do an activity used to suggest 20-30 minutes at least three times a week, but it is now being further suggested that due to our obesogenic environment, this figure requires adjustment to 30 minutes at least five times a week. I go further than this and get my client's to commit to doing some form of activity everyday for at least 30 minutes. This doesn't necessarily have to be exercise per se, but could just be changing some of your daily activities in order to increase your physical activity. For example, it could mean that you park further away in the car park, that you take the stairs instead of the escalator, and that you walk up to the next bus stop on your route to work. This will involve little time, but will have a huge affect over a week. It will help to use up some surplus energy instead of storing it all as fat.

As an example of how you could get started with a new activity, the following walking programme may be helpful. This can be graded really easily, takes you into the fresh air, and is easy on the joints. If you get together with a few friends, you will all soon begin to feel the benefit. To avoid any negative negotiation with yourself and the others of, "shall we shan't we," commit to going out even if it is pouring down with rain. (He made us waterproof!) Simply don your raincoat and your boots and just get out in the fresh air. It will stimulate, invigorate, get you fitter and recharge your batteries.

Beginners Walking Programme

Before starting, you will need to consider having:

o   Water bottles

o   Walking poles

o   Mobile phone

o   Suitable clothes, layers are best.

o   **Proper supportive footwear that offers a degree of shock absorbency. This is imperative for ALL physical activities.**

Whilst this appears like a list any boy scout would be proud of, the items are necessary if you want to take your activity seriously.

I have also included **F.I.T.T. (Frequency, Intensity, Time, Type)** principles into the following example that you may like to consider. These principles can be applied to planning any of your activities. I find the more I plan, the less excuses I am able to come up with, and this applies to both myself and my clients:

Frequency- How often are you going to walk?

Intensity- How hard and at what speed are you going to walk? Are you going to go up and down hills?

Walking can be split into three basic paces:

Level 1- Wandering, ambling, shopping pace

Level 2 - Active walking, striding, relaxed—but with purpose

Level 3 - Competitive walking, fast paced

Time – How long are you planning to walk?

Type – What are you going to do? Where are you going? How far are you going?

Walking Posture

Of equal importance is how you walk. Shuffling along with your shoulders hunched is not going to be entirely beneficial.

Pointers for good posture are:

• Think about growing tall from the top of your head pulling up through the spine as if you are trying to elongate it.

• Make sure your feet land heel to toe.

- Keep your shoulders relaxed, back, and opening up through your chest.

- Keep your tummy pulled in away from the waistband.

- When you walk, you swing your arms comfortably and push your elbows back behind you to help drive your walk.

- Keep your chin in and your neck relaxed.

Warming Up

Don't forget to warm up properly. Follow the guidelines outlined earlier on page 151. Include stretches if you can, especially if you are a beginner. Ten minutes taken warming up may save you much heartache later in avoiding things like pulled calf muscles. You will have a much better workout if you prepare properly.

Weekly Programme and Goals

The following example demonstrates how you can break down your group's goals to a weekly programme. This example is based around a 12-week SMART goal schedule (introduced on page 67) with FITT principles added. I have provided the first four-week schedules as an example.

Goals

Long Term:

S: We will be able to walk for 60 minutes at a low to moderate intensity without stopping to rest.

M: Yes, the goal is measurable as we will time ourselves.

A: Yes, the goal is achievable, and has been agreed with the group.

R: Yes, the goal is realistic as all members of the group walk a little.

T: The long term goal is time bound to 12 weeks.

Medium Term:

S: We will be be able to walk for 40 minutes at a low to moderate intensity without stopping to rest.

M: Yes, the goal is measureable as we will time ourselves.

A: Yes, the goal is achievable, and has been agreed with the group.

R: Yes, the goal is realistic.

T: The goal is time bound to 8 weeks.

Short Term:

S: We will be be able to walk for 30 minutes at a low to moderate intensity without experiencing fatigue.

M: Yes, the goal is measureable as above.

A: Yes, the goal is achievable, and has been agreed with the group.

R: Yes, the goal remains realistic.

T: The goal is time bound to 4 weeks.

Week 1:

F: 2 times a week

I: RPE 4-5 (Rate of perceived exertion)

T: 12-15 minutes

T: Walk on local road and park. Upon return, do flexibility exercises.

An end-of-the-week feedback session to discover how we all felt will help us plan for the following week's walking. If there is a setback or fatigue is hit sooner than anticipated, we will insert a short break.

Week 2

F: 2 times per week

I: RPE 4-5

T: 15 minutes

T: Walk on local road and park. Upon return, do flexibility exercises.

How do we all feel? The answer will help us plan for the following week's walking prescription. If there is a setback, we will plan accordingly.

Week 3

F: 2 times per week

I: RPE 4-5

T: 20 minutes

T: Walk on local road and park. Upon return, do flexibility exercises.

How do we all feel? Any problems? What can we do to get around these? The answers will help us plan the following week's walking. If there is a setback, we will plan accordingly.

Week 4

F: 2 times per week.

I: RPE 4-5

T: 30 minutes

T: Walk on local road and park. Upon return, do flexibility exercises.

   Was the short term goal achieved? If it wasn't, what were the reasons?

As the weeks progress you would, of course, slowly increase your time and effort, perhaps including a few hills. It is generally accepted that, if you are using FITT principles, that you just increase one of them at a time. This way you can ensure you are grading your activity sensibly. Of course, you also don't need to go to these extremes, and you can use this same formula as a guide. I just find that for both myself and my clients, if I have it all planned, I have already committed them and myself to the goals.

This is simply one idea among the thousands through which you could improve your heart and lung function. Have a look at Nordic Walking as an alternative . If walking isn't your thing, then look at the local classes that are available, think about swimming, or get together with people from your church and fellowship and organise activities yourselves. There are now a number of Christian football and netball leagues. It just takes a little organisation. There will be all sorts of activities and classes locally, perhaps have a look at:

o   Your local sports centre

o   Village hall notice boards

o   Local shop windows

o   Adult Education classes

o   Library

o   Local health clubs

o   Swimming pools

I am hoping that the above has provided you with at least some ideas as to how to get started on your cardiovascular fitness.

Muscular Strength and Endurance (MSE)

We have looked very briefly at how we can improve our **cardiovascular** system, and now we will have a look at **muscular strength and endurance (MSE)** as it applies to your musculoskeletal system. Very briefly, **muscular strength** is how much you can lift at any one time, and **muscular endurance** is how long the muscle can keep doing what you are asking of it. MSE is all about posture, movement, balance, and the ability of your muscles to perform the tasks you need them to. Also, the big muscles in your lower limbs possess valves, which assist the blood in your veins to return to the heart, often referred to as a secondary pump. Of course, all these systems work in synergy, and so in order to achieve **cardiovascular fitness**, you also need **MSE**.

If we consider **functional fitness in respect to MSE,** we will be thinking along these lines: How easy do I find carrying the shopping, mowing the lawn, lifting boxes, cutting the hedge, how long can I stand at work? This is the basic strength and endurance we need for our ADL's. Over and above that, if our muscles are toned, strong, and can do work for a reasonable amount of time without tiring, then we are going to get around more easily, have less aches and pains, and have improved posture. Just having good musculature does not, however, guarantee good posture, and we will consider this shortly. Resistance training, as it is often referred to, will challenge the body in a way that will increase the number of capillaries, and therefore, good blood flow in the muscles worked. It will also increase the number of mitochondria, which are involved in energy production, as well as the increasing density of the muscle tissue. I would like to look firstly at some very basic principles for improving both muscular strength and endurance, but before I do, I need to clear up one of the biggest myths that surrounds this subject:

Myth:

❑   Doing weights and weighted exercises causes big muscles

It is actually quite difficult to build substantial muscles. Again, it is all down to your genetics and body shape. Remember my client, the gentleman who wanted to put weight on to join the military. He would never, ever, ever, be able to build large muscles, unless he took lots of steroids, but that would probably kill him. There was not one little, dinky tiny gene in his body that would have helped him. He was an ectomorph and would be all his life. If I get a client that suggests they want to avoid weights for this reason, I usually explain it by saying that if they wanted to build muscle, then I would need them training six days a week, probably for two to three hours each day, to be on an extremely strict eating regime, and they would have to be lifting weights that neither of us could get off the floor. I exaggerate, but I need to get the message across that building large muscles is nearly impossible for most people.

You can really make these weighted and weight-bearing exercises work for you in any way you choose. It is all down to your specific programme. It is like moulding a piece of clay. So, again, it is all about what you want to achieve.

Exactly the same basic principles apply to improving MSE that apply to reaching **cardiovascular fitness**, that is, we need to overload the system.

We need to consider **SAID:**

Specific

Adaptation

Imposed

Demands

In other words, whatever you get your muscles to do, they will soon adapt, just like your heart and lungs did to the extra workload you are putting on them. It is a complete waste of your time, and probably your money, if you spend time working under your target levels. Your muscles and your heart and lungs will just be cruising, and you won't get any real fitness improvement or health benefit. This is partly the reason that many people give up after six weeks of a training programme. The body will have adjusted to whatever activity you are doing and will reach what we call a plateau. If you are trying to lose weight, with healthy eating and exercise, this is when you may well become despondent, as the fantastic early results you were achieving have now slowed right down. The answer to this is to keep challenging the body in a new way, such as, changing the activity, attending a harder class, or increasing the intensity. By adjusting your activity programme correctly, you can achieve whatever results you are after, but you need to keep fine tuning the programme. Personal trainers do this for you, and so will your gym staff at your local facility, so if you get stuck, ask. I will also provide my contacts at the end, so that you can always contact me.

How do I improve my MSE?

Just as you did for your cardiovascular activities, you need to establish what it is you want to achieve. Do you, for example, want to tone your legs, build your shoulders up, improve your posture, and/or flatten your tummy? It is about being specific and tailoring your exercises accordingly. I am going to suggest a few exercises to get you started, but firstly it might be helpful if I expand on the principle of **SAID** (**S**pecific, **A**daptation, **I**mposed, **D**emands).

We will now be referring to both **repetitions** and **sets.**

❖ **Repetitions** are the number of times you repeat that particular exercise in any one go.

❖ **Sets** are the number of times you repeat those **repetitions.**

For example, I can do 12 bicep curls, which is 12 **repetitions**. Then I pause for 30 seconds, and then I repeat them twice more. So I will have done 3 **sets** (a total of 36 bicep curls).

To Apply This:

Strength: If you want to build muscle as much as you can to become as strong as you can, then you need to lift heavy weights. They need to be so heavy that you can only lift them a small number of times, repetitions. This challenges the muscle in a way that increases the number and thickness of the muscle fibres.

Endurance: If, however, you want to work at building your endurance, then you need to lift lighter weights more often, so more repetitions. This will get your muscles to improve efficiency at maintaining work over a longer period of time.

For **general physical fitness improvement and toning**, you need to be thinking of somewhere between the two. The key to the weight you need to be using is to pick the one that you will fail to complete the 2nd or 3rd set, depending on what you want to achieve. For my own training, I use a weight that I can do reasonably, but hard to achieve: 12 repetitions in the 1st and 2nd sets. Then I want to be able to get to only about 8 - 10 repetitions in the 3rd set and fail. If I could easily complete this last set, then my weight is no longer heavy enough and my body will just be on tick over (idling). So, for general fitness, look at the middle column in the strength and endurance chart on the next page. This is the level I suggest you work at to start with.

Strength and Endurance Chart

Strength	General Fitness /Toning	Endurance
Heavy Weights	Weight to failure on 2nd to 3rd set	Weight will depend on what you are training for: swimming, athletics, etc.
Specific training regimes, such as pyramid, supers sets	Simpler basic routines	
Low number of sets and reps	Greater number of sets and reps	Sets and reps will again be tailored to what you are looking to achieve
Eg: 6- 8 Reps 1 - 2 Sets	Eg: 10-12 Reps (Beginners 8-12) 2-3 Sets (Beginners 1-2)	Eg: 12-15 Reps 2-3 + Sets May be performed faster than other formats depending on desired outcomes
Rest interval between sets will depend on programme used	Rest interval: 30secs - 60secs	Rest interval between sets will depend on programme used

Which Exercises?

When it comes to MSE activities, and especially if you have never done this sort of exercise previously, then I would suggest that you join a class that is at a suitable level for you. This way, you will learn proper technique and correct posture. Using fitness DVD's and books such as this one are all very well, but you don't get the feedback that you need. This is why we all have mirrors in our fitness studios, and not, as some people think, to do your make up! It is to enable the instructor and yourself to correct your form and technique.

Yoga???

It might be appropriate to mention here the question that often arises, as to which exercise classes may be appropriate for the Bible believing Christian. This is, of course, down to your own choice and the guidance that you have through your own spiritual walk. One such example that I get asked time and again is regarding yoga. There is a huge variety of opinion on this, and some Christians I know teach yoga?? Personally, I would not. **Yoga is Hindusim** - Period!! It doesn't matter how you dress it up or try to re-invent it or even make it "Christian Yoga" which I have seen advertised. Yoga focuses on the Kundalini spirit. So.....if you are asking yourself if you should participate in any form of yoga, have a look at where it comes from and look up Kundalini. Reflect back on our Bible studies. If you are not focusing on the one true God, then who or what are you mediating on?

Up until recently, I have been teaching Fitness Pilates, thinking that was a safer option. It is not!! In researching further regarding the origins of Pilates, I discover that its founder, a German called Joseph Pilates, drew much of his ideas from Zen and Yoga/ Hinduism and embraced these when designing his Pilates workouts. So, PLEASE BE AWARE!

Posture, Core Stability, and Strength

A basic concept of *all* physical activity is to improve your foundational **core stability and strength**. Whether you are walking, running, or simply sitting down, posture, core stability, and strength are key to safe and effective activity. Imagine them as being central to what you do. If you have good posture, which in turn is supported by good core stability and strength, then you are less likely to experience aches and pains.

Posture

The more you look, the more you see. Just have a look around where you are right now. If there is anyone close, just have a critical look at how they are sitting or standing. Are they rounding their shoulders, are they slouched, are they walking straight, do their knees come together as they move, or do their feet turn in? How many people do you know who have niggles (discomforts) and aches and pains in the back, the hips, the knees? Unfortunately, the modern day lifestyle doesn't lend itself to maintaining good posture and muscle balance. We sit down all day at computers or driving, leaning forwards and slouching. We don't move much, our muscles are out of condition, and if we don't work them and stretch them out, they will shorten.

The hamstrings, for example, run up and down the back of the leg. Their job is to flex the knee and extend the hip. If I sit a lot, especially for hours at a time, and don't condition these muscles and stretch them so that they are flexible, then they will effectively shorten up and, because of where they are attached, this will, in turn, pull on my lower spine and probably give me backaches.

Most of us have muscle imbalances and if these are extreme, they can easily cause much pain and discomfort. If you are getting a lot of pain, especially in the knees, backs, and hips, it may well be worth seeing someone like a sports injury specialist or physiotherapist. They would be able to assess your posture and movement and give you specific exercises to do which will help correct the problem. I have to do one-legged squats to correct a muscle imbalance in my right leg. If I don't do them and ensure that my right leg is going straight, then I get excruciating pain in my hips when I run.

So, don't accept that it is down to your age or that you are doing too much. Get to the bottom of why the pain is there and then do whatever you can to correct it. In many cases losing any extra weight you are carrying can also make a considerable difference to your joints

Whilst, as I have already mentioned, having a fitness or health professional correct your posture is preferable, here are some pointers towards improving your posture.

Standing in front of a full length mirror, check the following:

o   Where are your hands? Are they to the front of your legs or down the side? Ideally they need to be lying down by the side seam of your trousers. Gently ease your shoulders up, back, and then down. Put your hands down to the side.

o   Where is your chin? Is it sticking out? Bring it back in until it feels more comfortable.

o   How is your posture? Grow tall as if you are on sky hooks, lengthening up through the spine, without sticking your chin out. Feel your tummy tightening up as you do it.

o   Where is your tummy? Breathe out and pull your tummy in and away from your waistband.

o   Where are you feet? Are they turned in or out? Make sure your toes are in line with your heels, your heels in line with your knees, and your knees in line with your hips.

o   Where are your shoulders? Are they level? Just swing one arm backwards and forwards, really shaking it out for about 3 minutes. Has it become longer than the other one? Now do the other one and see if they are now level. If you tend to carry your bags on one shoulder only, or use one arm predominantly, then that side will carry much more tension in it. Swing that arm out to get rid of some of the tension.

Poor posture   **Improved posture**

Rounded shoulders   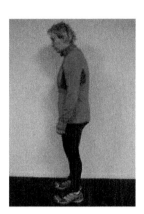   Shoulders back and down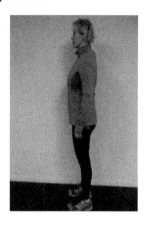

Head down   Head in line with spine

Collapsed spine   Elongated spine

Core Stability and Strength

Your core muscles are just that, your trunk muscles—the ones that support your spine —your abdominal muscles and the muscles around your shoulders, hips, and pelvis. I also include the deep pelvic floor muscles when considering the core muscles.

These muscles effectively wrap around the torso like a corset and, together, they stabilise and support the spine helping your balance and all movement. If these muscles are weak, then all other movement is likely to be out of line and poorly supported, and you are more likely to suffer from symptoms such as back pain. As an example, think for a minute about someone who has a physically demanding job: bending, lifting heavy weights, and carrying. Think of the movement that this involves: bending over, then lifting a heavy weight which, in turn, puts a huge amount of stress on the lower spine. If this person's core muscles are weak and out of condition, then you can imagine that there is nothing to support the lifting. Again, if you are sitting all day, your core muscles will be weak and your hamstrings tight, which will put a vast amount of strain on your joints and especially your back.

What Can I Do to Strengthen My Core and Give Me a Flat Tummy and a Six Pack?

The bad news is that simply doing lots of sit ups will neither strengthen your core muscles or flatten your stomach. You also need to be working off the calories to get rid of the layers of fat that lay over the muscles. The good news is that the following exercises will provide a basic routine with the aim of getting you started, which will begin to tone you up as well as provide vital strength and stability to all the important core muscles.

I also suggest that you try and attend a class or gym with fully qualified instructors that will ensure you learn the correct technique.

Basic Core Exercises

i. The Pre-Plank

- Lie face down on the floor with your face resting on your hands.
- Relax into the floor.
- Breathe out and draw your tummy up to meet your spine.
- Try not to use any other muscles other than your tummy.

If lying down is awkward, then an alternative is to stand upright with your back against a wall. Breathe out and pull your tummy in and away from the waistband.

ii. The Pre-Half Plank

- When you have mastered the pre-plank and can feel your abdominal muscles contracting, come up onto all fours.
- First, arch your back up like a cat stretch.
- Second, let your back sag right down.
- Third allow your back to relax in the middle of these extremes. This is called neutral alignment and is the shape your back is when you are standing, following its natural curvature.
- And now repeat the above exercise.

Breath out and pull your stomach in to meet the spine.

Again, try and work the abdominal muscles on their own.

Natural spine
Pull the tummy muscles in towards
the back whilst breathing out.

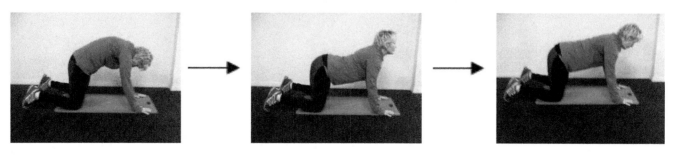

This exercise is progressed gradually as you become stronger. If you feel any tension in your lower spine, then you need to drop back to the previous level.

Here are the next two levels:

iii. The Half Plank

- Return to lying on the floor face down.

- Bend your elbows and place them out in front of you, just in front of the shoulders.

- Now you are going to repeat the above exercise, breathe out and pull your tummy in to meet the spine.

- Only this time, you are also going to lift your bottom off the floor, not too high.

You need a gentle slope down from your head. You are resting on the padded bit just above your knee, not on the knee joint itself. Your tummy is doing all the work. **Don't forget to breathe**.

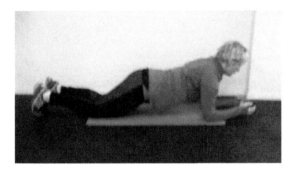

Half plank

iv. The Full Plank

Still further progression is to lift up onto your toes instead of your knees.

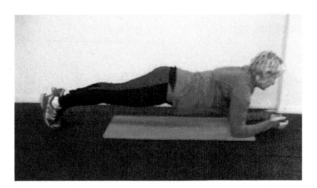

Full plank

All the same principles apply. Keep your head in line with the spine and tummy pulled in. Breathe normally.

Try and avoid the following:

Avoid: Lifting your bottom too high. You need it to be level with your head.

Avoid: Looking down. Eyeball just in front of you to keep your head in line with the spine.

Avoid: Using your shoulders to take all the weight instead of focusing the effort on your abdominals.

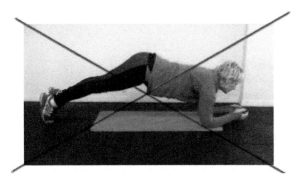 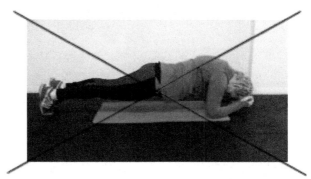

All of the above plank exercises can be held for as long as you can maintain the correct technique. To start with, it may well be literally seconds. If you can hold each exercise for a minute, then it is time to move on to the next level. At the same time, **watch your backs**. It is a bit of a chicken and an egg scenario, as you want to strengthen your abdominals in order to better support your spine, but you don't want to hurt your spine in doing so. If you feel any pressure at all on the lower spine, you must finish the exercise and return to the floor.

There exists a vast range of core stability and strengthening exercises that you can find online and in books. Try and find a local exercise class to join. Especially if you are doing sports, core conditioning classes can be extremely beneficial. I teach a class that is based on the large physiotherapy fitness balls. It is hard work but effective.

Here are a few more basic exercises to get you thinking about your core muscles:

v. The Superman

- Start off on all fours, with a leg at each back corner and your hands aligned under you shoulders.
- Correct your spine so that it is neutral alignment (as it is when you are standing, with its natural curvature).
- Pull your tummy in to meet the spine (as in the above exercises) without moving the spine itself.
- Keeping your head in line with your spine, extend one arm out and the opposite leg behind you: superman.

- You are focusing on lengthening through your spine whilst keeping your hips level.

- Slowly and controlled, change the arm and leg to the opposite ones.

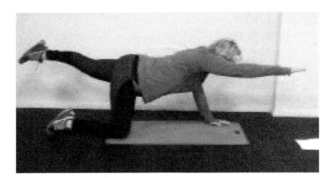

Superman

vi. The Standing Superman

The Standing superman is the next progression.

Make sure your shoulders and hips stay level.

The Superman is all about stabilising the torso/core.

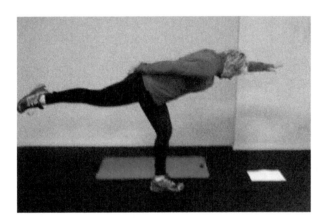

Standing Superman

vii. The Back Roll

It is suggested that if you are new to this exercise, stand up against a wall, which helps to guide you.

- Breathe out and pull your tummy in away from your waistband.

- Grow tall and lengthen through the spine, chin in.

- Slowly roll your chin to your chest and then follow it down by rolling your back forwards.

- Allow you shoulders and arms to relax.

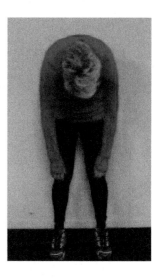

- Allow your back to relax whilst keeping your stomach muscles pulled in to support it.

- Relax and take this exercise *only* as far as you feel comfortable.

- Slowly uncurl, using your core muscles to straighten you up.

- As you progress this exercise, it is possible to stand away from the wall.

Basic Abdominal Exercises

Again, there are a million and one exercises that will work the abdominal muscles. The key, however, is in working them correctly. The following exercises are an attempt to ensure correct technique and to give a few pointers as to how to make your exercises both safe and effective. To illustrate how easy it is to get it wrong, I will use the following exercise. You may have seen people executing a sit up with their feet anchored under a bench or with someone holding their feet. If you are aware of what you are doing and know how to correctly contract your abdominal muscles, then this exercise can have some beneficial effect. BUT, if you don't, then the chances are you will use your leg muscles and hip flexors instead of your abdominals to perform the sit up.

Sit Up With Feet Anchored

To prepare:

- Lie on your back with your spine relaxed in its natural curve, in neutral spine.

- Bend your knees with your feet on the floor or resting on your heels.

- Engage the muscles that you were using in the above exercises—that is all your lower abdominal muscles—and if you know where your pelvic floor muscles are, pull them in as well.

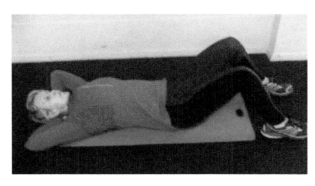

Sit up with feet anchored

If you have spent a few weeks practicing the plank every day, you will by now, hopefully, be able to flatten your tummy quite well. If you still need to lose the fat on top, then don't despair. Instead try and be aware of how well you are now contracting those deep muscles, and you should still be able to pull your tummy in quite nicely. These are your basic anchoring muscles. You need to keep them contracted and your tummy flat as we add on some further abdominal work.

i. The Basic Sit Up

- Prepare as above and place your hands at the base of your thighs.

- Imagine, and this is really important, a large piece of elastic that stretches from your rib cage down to your pelvic girdle. If that bit of elastic contracts and shortens, then the two ends, your head end and bottom end, will want to come together and bend in the middle. This is going to make you perform a sit up and NOT by pulling and yanking on your head.

- So, LEAVE YOUR HEAD ALONE.

- Breathe out, contract your Rectus Abdominus (imagine someone is going to punch you in the tummy), and slide your hands up your legs.

- It doesn't matter how far you lift, but it does matter that your tummy is doing all the work.

- Until your abdominal muscles begin to tighten up, you may well feel tension in your shoulders and the back of your neck. If you do, relax, and then start again.

- Once you have accomplished this, place your fingers to your temples and repeat the exercise.

- Try and keep your chin away from your chest.

- Repeat 12-15 repetitions and 2-3 sets.

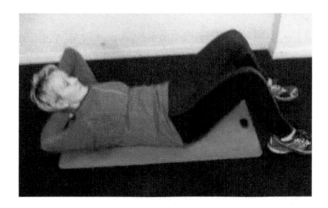

Basic sit up

ii. The Obliques (Side Tummy Muscles)

Using the same principle as the above exercise now, we can apply this in working the Obliques, which help

you to rotate and turn your torso.

- Prepare as in the above exercise.

- This time instead of sliding the hands up the legs, cross your hands over as you sit up and reach down
  the side of the opposite leg, so that you are turning to the side as you lift.

- Repeat 12-15 repetitions and 2-3 sets

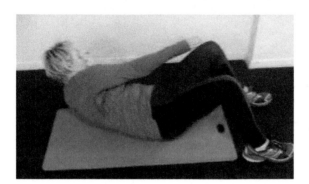

Obliques

Basic Back Exercises

Part of the core musculature are the back muscles. All muscles work in groups, some lengthening, whilst

the ones opposite are shortening. The core muscles of the abdominal region and the back work in synergy with

each other. If muscles are not worked equally, then imbalances may occur. Therefore it is just as important to

have strong and stable spinal muscles as it is to have strong core muscles.

i The Uside-Down Sit Up

This next exercise is like an upside down sit up and I prefer to work it using a fit ball, but it can be done on

the floor without one. Fit balls are available at all the discount stores these days and cost you very little. They

open up a vast range of core training exercises and are fantastic for anyone with arthritis or weak joints as you

can use the ball to support you. Just sitting on the ball will challenge both your balance and core.

- Curl yourself over the ball and relax, stretching the back.

- You need to place your feet and knees firmly on the floor to avoid slipping back when you perform the
  lift.

- Now place your fingers to you temples and using your back muscles, raise your shoulders off the ball.

- Try not to tip your head back, and keep it in line with your spine.

- Repeat 12-15 repetitions and 2-3 sets.

Hyperextensions on the floor

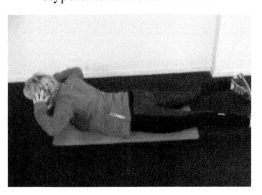

Or off the fit ball

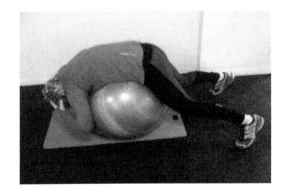
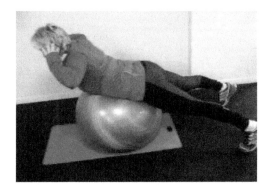

Having now established where and what your core muscles do, continue to bear these in mind as we look at some **Basic Muscular Strength and Endurance Exercises.** Your core muscles need to be working at all times in order to support and stabilise you as you perform the following exercises. You need to be challenging the body whilst at the same time working within your own limits. If you know that you are weak in a certain area, then be sensible about it and use the easiest version of the exercise until you strengthen up, or indeed miss it altogether. The following exercises are simply to help you get started. Remember that your body will soon adapt to the new regime and again I suggest that you seek out a class or attend a gym if you really want to see results. Using equipment will add another dimension to your exercises and will provide for a wider variety. I use elastic fitness tubes, similar to a skipping rope, but you can use them for weighted exercises. And, as mentions, I also use the fit ball. Both of these can be easily obtained inexpensively. They often come with exercise sheets and are a great addition to your repertoire.

Basic muscular strength and endurance exercises: Arms

i. Push Ups

The push up is what is termed a compound exercise. In other words, it works a lot of muscles for the price of one exercise. It works all the muscles around your shoulders, your arm muscles (front and back, upper and lower), your leg muscles (for the full push up), and your core muscles. I love this exercise!

The best bit is that you can grade a push up so that everyone can do it:

Push up Level 1 - I use two push ups as alternatives at this level.

The Wall Push Up

- Pull your tummy muscles in away from your waistband as in your core exercises.

- Stand about arms length away from the wall.

- Now place your hands just over shoulder width apart on the wall.

- Lean towards the wall.

- Bend your elbows until your nose is almost touching the wall.

- Straighten your arms up again without locking your elbows out.

- Repeat 12-15 repetitions and 2-3 sets.

If you have weak wrists, try using your fist rather than your hand onto the wall as this keeps it straighter and puts it under less pressure.

Push Up with the Ball

This is an exercise I use if people have, say, arthritis in their shoulders as the ball can be used to take as much weight as you need.

- Lie on the ball on your stomach and then move progressively further forward, so that the ball is placed further and further down your legs. As you move out, you will feel that more and more weight is being added to your shoulders. When you feel that this is enough, stop, and this is then your push up position. For Level 1, this can be as close to the ball as you need for the extra support.

- Keeping your abdominals tightly in, bend you elbows until your nose is just hovering off the floor.

- Straighten your arms without locking your elbows.

- Repeat 12-15 repetitions and 2-3 sets.

Push up Level 2

Push Up with the Box

From the Level 1 push up, progression is all a question of weight transfer.

For the basic push up, start with the Box.

- Start on all fours with your knees hip distance apart and your hands placed slightly wider than shoulder width.

- Pulling your abdominal muscles in, bend your elbows until your nose is just off the floor.

- Straighten your arms again without locking your elbows.

- Repeat 12-15 repetitions and 2-3 sets.

Push up Level 3

The Three-Fourth Push Up

Exactly the same as the box push up, this has transferred the body weight forward slightly so that there is more weight going onto the push up.

- Take care to keep the abdominal muscles in tightly to support the back.

- The push up itself is executed exactly the same as the above.

- Repeat 12-15 repetitions and 2-3 sets.

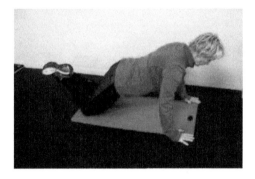

The three-fourth push up

Push up Level 4

The Full Push Up

More weight has now been transferred onto the chest and shoulders area and you are now working against a considerable amount of your body weight.

- Take care to keep the abdominal muscles in tightly to support the back. It is the Plank, but with moving parts.

- The push up itself is executed exactly the same as the above.

- Repeat 12-15 repetitions and 2-3 sets.

The full push up (level 4)

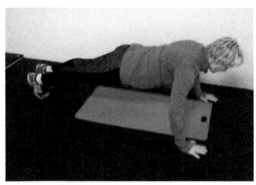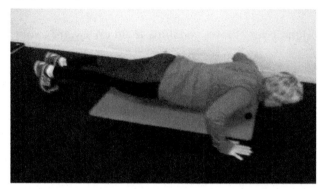

You have already worked the arm muscles in the push up, but if you want to try a few more arm exercises, here are a few to have a go at.

ii. The Bicep Curl

Use a fit tube, or cans of beans! The beauty about using a tubey is that you can alter the amount of resistance you work with. By standing with your feet wider apart you can make it harder, or bringing your feet in or using just one foot, you can make things easier. Key to this exercise is keeping your abdominals in tight so that the pressure of the lift is not on your back. You will find that you can really feel your tummy working.

- Stand on your tubing, with a handle in each hand. You don't have to grip the handles, a gentle hold with an open hand is adequate.

- Place your feet at a distance whereby you feel the resistance, but not so much that you can't bend your arm.

- Pull your abdominals in to support your stance and back.

- Bend your elbows and curl your arms up to meet the shoulders. Try to keep the wrist straight and your elbows in to your side as you lift.

- Straighten your arm back out without locking the elbows out.

- Repeat 12-15 repetitions and 2-3 sets.

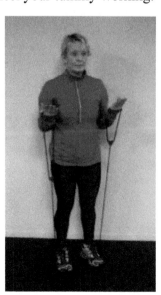

Bicep curl

iii. The Upright Row

This exercise works a number of muscles in the back and the shoulder joint. Again, it will also mean that you have to work your abdominals to support your stance and back.

Using the tubey again, take up your start position standing on the tubey as you did for the bicep curl.

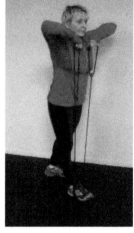

- This time you need to place your thumbs together in front of you with your arms down and straight (elbows very slightly bent).

- Bend your elbows and draw them up towards your ears. Try and keep the thumbs as close to each other as you can. As if you are zipping yourself up.

- Repeat 12-15 repetitions and 2-3 sets.

Upright row

iv. Dips

Having worked the front of the arm in the bicep curl, this exercise will target your tricep muscle, the underarm muscle.

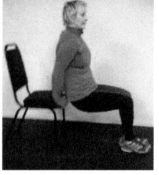

- Find yourself a sturdy chair or use a third step on the staircase.

- Sit on it.

- Place your hands over the lip and launch your bottom just off the edge. Ideally you should have your knees at about right angles.

- Now bend at your elbow and lower your bottom straight down to the floor.

- Straighten at your elbow and return to your start position without locking your elbows.

- Repeat 12-15 repetitions and 2-3 sets.

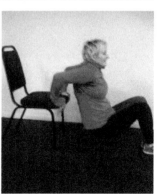

Dips

Basic muscular strength and endurance exercises: Legs

i. The Squat

This exercise works a number of muscles in the leg, the front, back and gluteus, your behind, and your hip flexors as well as your core stabilising muscles. This exercise can help towards strengthening and stabilising both the hip and knee joints as it works the muscles surrounding them.

This is a tricky one to coach even when you are standing in front of your client, so in order to get the technique as close as we can without me seeing you, grab yourself a chair.

Squat

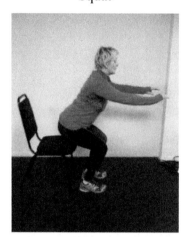

- Stand approximately 6 inches in front of the chair with your back to the chair as if you are going to sit on it.

- Have your toes in line with your ankles, in line with your knees, in line with your hips.

- Grow tall through the top of your head and pull your abdominals in tight.

- Now bend at the knee and brush the chair with your behind.

- Straighten up again without locking your knees out.

- Allow your back to relax and let it do what it normally does when you sit down. It will bend forward slightly from the hip. It is supported by your core muscles.

- Repeat 12-15 repetitions and 2-3 sets.

If this is too difficult, you don't have to go down as far as the chair. Alternatively, try using a fit ball again:

- Stand against a wall with the ball in the small of your back.

- Stand upright to start and pull your abdominals in tight.

- Take one step in front of you with your feet still hip-distance apart.

- Bend your knees and allow the ball to roll with you.

- Straighten back up again without locking the knees.

- Repeat 12-15 repetitions and 2-3 sets.

ii. The Squat With Side Leg Raise.

If you want to expand on this exercise, try adding in a side leg raise, but maintain the squat.

- Take up your start position as above.

- Perform a downward squat as above.

- On the up phase raise one leg to the side. The key here is to keep the toes pointing to the front in order to target the side leg muscles.

- Lower the leg again as you return to the squat. You can alternate legs or do a complete set on one side and then change legs.

- Repeat 12-15 repetitions and 2-3 sets on each leg.

ii. Lunges

Again for the legs. This one changes the muscles that are being used slightly and is a good basic exercise to incorporate into your routine.

Lunge

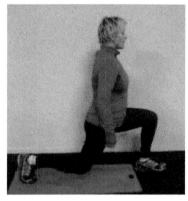

- Standing up straight with your abdominals pulled in. Take a stride forward, keeping one foot far in front of the other.

- Your front knee needs to remain behind the toes. Otherwise when you perform the exercise, it will put a lot of strain through your knee joint.

- Bend the back knee straight down towards the floor, as if you were going to kneel, but don't let the knee touch the floor.

- Straighten back up and keep the feet in place.

- Try and avoid any forward movement in this exercise. You are simply taking the back knee straight down as far as is comfortable.

- Repeat 12-15 repetitions and 2-3 sets. Change legs and repeat. You can alternate the sets, one leg then the other.

Power and Speed Exercises

If I was writing a book aimed at athletes and sports specialists, then these elements of physical fitness would be invaluable. I am anticipating that this is not who will be reading this book and so I am omitting the intricacies of training for speed and power.

Mobility and Flexibility Exercises

We have already discussed briefly the advantages of maintaining mobility (the normal range of movement) and of developing our flexibility to improve posture and avoid injuries and aches pains. Ideally, there is no better place to learn these than in a class format, which you will now be tired of hearing me say. The following few exercises are what are called developmental stretches, that is, they help to improve your flexibility.

There are a number of key facts that you need to consider when performing these exercises:

- It is **vital** that your muscles are warm when you perform these exercises to avoid injury. The warmer they are, the easier they will be to work.

- Your muscles need to be as relaxed as they can be in order to perform these exercises optimally. It is not a good idea to try and stretch muscles that are under a lot of tension.

- You need time to stretch properly. Each stretch needs to be held from 30-45 seconds and not rushed.

- Try and work with the muscles and not against them.

i. The Hamstring Stretch.

There are various ways of performing a stretch for this muscle. The best one for you will be the one that you can feel working, but that is also comfortable to hold, so that you can allow yourself to stretch. Many people find this one in particular rather awkward to achieve, especially if you are not very flexible. I have, therefore, chosen two that most people find they are capable of doing.

- For the first one you need to find a bench to sit on: picnic tables are great for this one. It needs to be a hard surface, so I'm afraid the settee (couch) won't work. (I use our kitchen table.)

- Place the leg you are going to stretch first on the surface and just let the other one stay on the floor.

- Sit up tall and pull your abdominals in.

- Bend straight forwards over your stretching leg, but aim to reach your toes with your chin, rather than just collapsing through the lower back. If this feels awkward, grab a towel or strap and hook it over your foot and pull gently towards you whilst remaining in a sitting position.

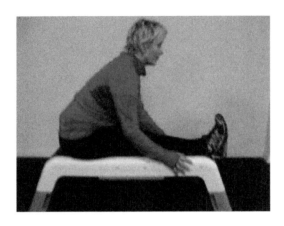

Hamstring stretch

- Try and keep your knee down on the supporting surface.

- After about 20 seconds, ease yourself out of the stretch. Bend the knee and relax it and then go straight down into the stretch again, holding it for a further 30 seconds. Try and see if you can extend the stretch.

- Repeat with the other leg.

The Alternate Hamstring Stretch

If this exercise is just too awkward for you, try this variation:

- Sit on a chair with the leg you want to stretch out in front, the toes curled up towards your shin.

- Have the other knee bent with your foot firmly on the floor.

- Sit up tall and pull your abdominals in tightly.

- Again, you can use a towel or strap around the ball of your foot.

- Keep your back straight and lean towards this leg.

- Hold the stretch as in the above exercise and repeat accordingly.

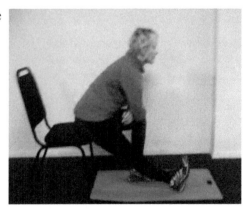

Alternate hamstring stretch

ii. The Hip Flexor and Quadricep Stretch

This exercise is often used to stretch these muscles (the front of leg and the flexors that lift the leg). My version is an alternative that isn't quite so hard on the knee joint angle.

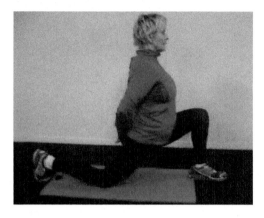

Hip flexor and Quad stretch

- Grab a chair for support and have cushion handy for your knee to rest on.
- Stand up tall and pull your abdominals in.
- Grow tall and take a stride out with one leg in front.
- Using the chair for support, slowly lower the back knee to the floor and the cushion.
- You are looking for a slope back from thigh to knee on the back leg to stretch the required muscles out.
- The front knee wants to be at a comfortable open angle of not less than 90 degrees.
- Keep your torso upright and your shoulders back.
- Hold for 30-40 seconds and then ease up and change legs.

iii. The Calf Stretch

The best place to stretch your calf is off a step, preferably with a rail to hold onto.

- Stand with both feet firmly on the step, hip width apart and in line.
- Take the leg to be stretched and place the ball of the foot on the edge of the step.
- Now ease the heel down until you feel the calf stretching.
- Hold this for about 20 seconds, ease out of the stretch and then repeat for a hold of about 30 seconds.
- Change legs and repeat.

If you don't have a step handy;

- Lean your hands against a wall.

- Step one leg out behind.

- Lean into the wall until you feel the stretch in the back leg and repeat the stretches as above.

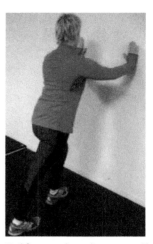

Calf stretch using a wall

iv. Triceps and Shoulder Stretch

This exercise is easier to describe by way of illustration rather than description.

- Place one hand on the opposite shoulder loosely.

- Use the opposite hand on the elbow to ease the arm past the shoulder and hold where you feel the stretch.

- Hold for 20 seconds, ease out of the stretch and then repeat and hold for about 30 seconds.

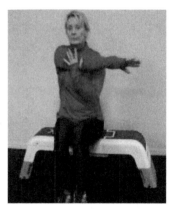

Triceps and shoulder stretch

v. Back Stretch

- For this stretch you need to be lying down with your knees bent.

- Gently pull your knees up to your chest and give them a hug.

- If you want to increase the stretch a little, take your head up to your knees, so you are rolled up like a hedgehog.

- You can roll gently around on the base of your spine and gently massage it out.

- Unroll gently.

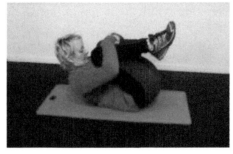

Back stretch

vi. Hip Stretch

- Whilst you are lying down and with your knees still bent, place one leg over the other knee at just above the ankle joint.

- To increase the stretch at the hip, ease the stretching leg away from you by pushing gently just below the knee joint.

- Alternatively, raise the supporting foot off the floor.

- Hold for about 20 seconds, ease out of the stretch and repeat and hold for about 30 seconds before changing legs.

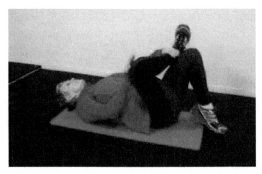 Hip stretch

And finally, as far as stretches go, use the fitness ball, if you have one, just to lie on and ease your back. Allow the ball to take your weight and just relax onto it. Whilst you are doing the above stretches, it might be an idea to put on some relaxing music and use the time to also unwind a little.

This concludes this chapter on physical activity and, indeed, the workbook. I am hoping that it has been of some help, at least in getting you started and in helping you see things from a different perspective. Commit all you do to Him and He will guide you every step of the way. You may well not agree with everything I have written, which is as it should be. Use your discernment to question and discuss the topics and come to your own understanding. This has been simply an introduction, and you may have many questions. To this end, please, do not hesitate to get in touch with me at the following e-mail address:

CuttingLooseContact@gmail.com

And Finally...

"For this reason, I fall on my knees before the Father, from whom every family in heaven and on earth receives its character. I pray that from the treasures of His glory He will empower you with inner strength by His Spirit, so that the Messiah may live in your hearts through your trusting. Also I pray that you will be rooted and founded in love, so that you, with all God's people, will be given strength to grasp the breadth, length, height and depth of the Messiah's love, yes, to know it, even though it is beyond all knowing, so that you will be filled with all the fullness of God.

Now to Him who by His power working in us is able to do far beyond anything we can ask or imagine, to Him be glory in the Messianic Community and in the Messiah Yeshua from generation to generation forever. Amen.

Ephesians 3:14-21

Author's website:

www.christianhealthandfitnessfellowship.co.uk

Please get in touch
with your feedback and questions:

CuttingLooseContact@gmail.com

I am available for:
workshops, presentations, and talks.

REFERENCES AND BIBLIOGRAPHY

Books and Articles

A Guide to Personal Fitness Training, Aerobics and Fitness Association of America, AFAA, California, 1997.

Barasi, M.E., *Human Nutrition. A health perspective.* 2nd edition, Hodder Arnold, Spain, 2003.

Borg, Gunner A.V. "Psychophysical Bases of Perceived Exertion," *Medicine and Science in Sports and Exercise,* 1982 (Vol. 14, No. 5, pp. 377– 381).

Collins, Williams, *English Dictionary. Complete and unabridged,* 6th edition, HarperCollins, Glasgow, 2003.

Obesity and Diabetes Management Certificate. Resource Manual, Level 4, Weight Management Centre, Tooting, WMC, 2009.

Seeley, R. R., Stephens, T.D., and Tate, P., *Anatomy and Physiology*, 6th edition, McGraw Hill. Boston, 2003

Stern, David H. *The Complete Jewish Bible.* Jewish New Testament Publications, Inc., Clarksville, Maryland, 1998.

Websites
(All accessed 02.2016.)

American College of Sports Medicine: http://www.acsm.org

Arthritis Research: http://www.arthritisresearchuk.org

Eating Disorders Help:

   Christian based: http://www.helenawilkinson.co.uk

   Secular based: Overeaters Anonymous: http://www.oagb.org.uk

Menopause and women's issues: Dr Marilyn Glenville PhD, available at: http://www.marilynglenville.com

Multiple Sclerosis Society: http://www.mstrust.org.uk

Multiple Sclerosis Trust: https://mssociety.org.uk

World Health Organisation (2014) www.who.int

CUTTING LOOSE

is available at:

olivepresspublisher.com

amazon.com

barnesandnoble.com

christianbook.com

deepershopping.com

and other online stores

Store managers:

Order wholesale through:

Ingram Book Company or

Spring Arbor

or by emailing:

olivepressbooks@gmail.com

Author's email and website:

CuttingLooseContact@gmail.com

christianhealthandfitnessfellowship.co.uk

Lightning Source UK Ltd.
Milton Keynes UK
UKOW07f0633210617
303730UK00011B/64/P

9 781941 173206